Pharmaceutical Ethics

Pharmaceutical Ethics

Edited by

Sam Salek

Welsh School of Pharmacy Centre for Socioeconomic Research,
University of Wales, Cardiff, UK

Andrew Edgar

Centre for Applied Ethics, Philosophy Section,
University of Wales, Cardiff, UK

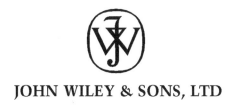

JOHN WILEY & SONS, LTD

Other Wiley Editorial Offices

John Wiley & Sons Inc., 111 River Street, Hoboken, NJ 07030, USA

Jossey-Bass, 989 Market Street, San Francisco, CA 94103-1741, USA

Wiley-VCH Verlag GmbH, Boschstr. 12, D-69469 Weinheim, Germany

John Wiley & Sons Australia Ltd, 33 Park Road, Milton, Queensland 4064, Australia

John Wiley & Sons (Asia) Pte Ltd, 2 Clementi Loop #02-01,
Jin Xing Distripark, Singapore 129809

John Wiley & Sons Canada Ltd, 22 Worcester Road, Etobicoke, Ontario, Canada M9W 1L1

Library of Congress Cataloging-in-Publication Data

Pharmaceutical ethics/edited by Sam Salek, Andrew Edgar.
        p. cm.
    Includes bibliographical references and index.
    ISBN 0-471-49057-1 (alk. paper)
        1. Pharmaceutical ethics. I. Salek, Sam. II. Edgar, Andrew.

    RS1005 .P475 2002
    174'.2—dc21

                                            2002071352

British Library Cataloguing in Publication Data

A catalogue record for this book is available from the British Library

ISBN 0 471 49057 1

Typeset in 10/12pt Palatino by Kolam Information Services Pvt. Ltd, Pondicherry India.
Printed and bound in Great Britain by Biddles Ltd, Guildford and King's Lynn
This book is printed on acid-free paper responsibly manufactured from sustainable forestry in
which at least two trees are planted for each one used for paper production.

Contents

Contributors

Mia Bauer *Statoil, Bergen, Norway.* E-mail: mbauer@statoil.no

Roger Bolton *Director of Scientific and Technical Policy, AstraZeneca R&D, Mereside 26T33, Alderley Park, Macclesfield, Cheshire SK10 4TG, UK.* E-mail: roger.bolton@astrazeneca.com

J. Lyle Bootman *Dean, and Professor of Pharmacy, Medicine and Public Health, College of Pharmacy, The University of Arizona, 1703 E. Mabel, Rm 344, Tucson, AZ 85721, USA*

Olivier Chassany *Direction de la Politique Médicale de l'Assistance Publique— Hôpitaux de Paris, Délégation Régionale à la Recherche Clinique, Carré Historique de l'hôpital Saint-Louis, 1 Avenue Claude Vellefaux, 75475 Paris Cedex 10, France.* E-mail: olivier.chassany@sls.ap-hop-paris.fr

Ruud Dessing *Apotheek AAN ZEE, Parallelboulevard 214A, 2202 HT Noordwijk, The Netherlands.* E-mail: ruud.dessing@xs4all.nl

Martin Duracinsky *Department of Internal Medicine, Saint-Louis University Hospital, 75010 Paris, France*

Andrew Edgar *Centre for Applied Ethics, Philosophy Section, University of Wales, P.O. Box 94 Colum Drive, Cardiff CF1 3XB, UK.* E-mail: edgar@cf.ac.uk

Chris Good Consultant Pharmaceutical Physician *Spinney Cottage, Thicket Grove, Maidenhead, Berks SL6 4LW, UK.* E-mail: chris.good@three-stacks.demon.co.uk

Amy J. Grizzle *Assistant Director, Center for Health Outcomes and PharmacoEconomic Research, University of Arizona, College of Pharmacy, Tucson, AZ 85721, USA*

David Hamilton *Department of Adult and Continuing Education, University of Glasgow, Scotland, UK.* E-mail: d.hamilton@admin.gla.ac.uk

Ivor Harrison   *Director, MSc in Regulatory Affairs, 8 Crystal Avenue, Heath, Cardiff CF2 5QJ, UK*

Sam Larsson   *Department of Social Work, University of Stockholm and Karlinska Institute, Center for Dependency Disorders, Magnus Huss Clinic, Stockholm, Sweden.* E-mail: sam.larsson@socarb.su.se

John Lilja   *Department of Biochemistry and Pharmacy, Abo Akademi University, Box 66, FIN-20521 Abo, Finland.* E-mail: johnlilja@hotmail.com

Isabelle Mahé   *Department of Internal Medicine, Lariboisière University Hospital, 75010 Paris, France*

Jon Merrills   *Consultant in Legal and Pharmaceutical Matters, Parkdale House, Peveril Drive, The Park, Nottingham NG7 1DE, UK.* E-mail: jonmerrils@compuserve.com

Jan Payne   *Institute for Human Studies in Medicine, First Medical Faculty, Charles University, Karlovo náměsti 40, 128 0 Prague 2, Czech Republic.* E-mail: jan.payne@lfl.cuni.cz

Sam Salek   *Director, Welsh School of Pharmacy Centre for Socioeconomic Research, University of Wales, Redwood Building, King Edward VII Avenue, Cardiff CF10 3XF, UK.* E-mail: salekss@cf.ac.uk

Roger Walker   *Director of Pharmaceutical Public Health, Gwent Health Authority, Mamhilad Park Estate, Pontypool, Gwent NP4 0YP, UK.* E-mail: roger.walker@gwent-ha.wales.nhs.uk

Preface

Over the last two or three decades, there has been an enormous growth in what is known as applied ethics. Academic moral philosophers devoted more and more of their time to considering, not abstruse issues of ethical language or reasoning, but moral problems as they occurred in the real world. In co-operation with professionals from various walks of life, and not least medicine, they explored the pressing moral issues that confronted those professionals in their everyday practice. Moral philosophers thus found a new role, not as sages who could resolve moral problems, but rather as experts on how professionals might deal with their own moral dilemmas: how they could be formulated and discussed; the sort of conceptual and argumentative resources one might be able to appeal to in order to make sense of and resolve those problems.

Medical ethics has long been a major part of applied ethics. However, pharmaceutical ethics has, perhaps, been rather neglected. There has been much sniping at the activities of commercial pharmaceutical companies. This has at times no doubt contained just criticism, but at other times was ill-formed and misguided. However, there has been relatively little material that sought to engage with people who were working in pharmacy and pharmacology, that was sympathetic to their perspectives and that addressed their everyday professional concerns. We hope that this collection of articles begins to stake out pharmaceutical ethics, not just as a field independent from medical ethics, but as a field that has the practitioner's perspective and concerns at its core.

The topics covered in this collection include general discussions of the nature of moral argument and moral decision-making, alongside responses to quite specific and concrete problems. After introductory chapters on ethical theory and the relationship between theory and real life decision-making, the first part of the book is concerned with a series of issues that the research pharmacist may confront, not least when conducting trials with human subjects. The concept of informed consent, that is so important in legal as well as ethical thought, receives detailed attention. The later part of the book is concerned with the moral and political problems that emerge from considering the use of pharmaceuticals in the wider society. In modern health care systems, questions of the cost and benefit of medicines cannot be avoided. The determination of the more appropriate ways to distribute pharmaceuticals and to reward their producers are not simply economic questions. They are questions about the moral and political presupposition that shape our assessment of the value of a pharmaceutical product to the patient and to society as a whole; they are questions about the justice of any given mechanism for distributing and promoting medicines.

The collection has drawn together contributors from throughout Europe and from the United States, and who collectively bring with them a wide range of experiences, both from within and outside of the pharmaceutical industry and pharmaceutical research. It is hoped that the collection will therefore appeal, not just to academics, but to anyone who is interested in the production and use of pharmaceuticals in contemporary society, be they established pharmaceutical scientists, pharmacy and medical practitioners, students just entering the profession, or interested lay persons – who, at the end of the day, are the beneficiaries (or otherwise) of the moral decisions that are made within the profession.

Sam Salek
BPharm, Phd, RPH, Hon MFPM
Andrew Edgar
BA, MA, DPhil

Foreword

Society has a right to expect that those who administer healthcare conform to the highest principles of ethical conduct and behaviour in their dealings with patients and those who care for them.

Defining these ethical standards across a broad range of cultural, religious and ethical communities has been a challenge to those organisations who operate globally, not least the international research-based pharmaceutical industry.

During the latter part of the 20th century, we witnessed the establishment of codes of practice for widely different activities such as the use of animals in medical research, the conduct of volunteer studies, clinical trials and the promotion of medicines. These codes of practice have established yardsticks against which to judge the quality of performance of healthcare professionals and the organisations in which they are employed; whether academic, industrial or government.

Across these various fields of pharmaceutical ethics, there has been a recurring dilemma as to how to establish objective, informed and intelligent debate and procedures of review between what inevitably is a very disparate community of concern. Ensuring that the voices that are heard in the discussions on pharmaceutical ethics are representative of the "stakeholders" will remain the subject of discussion; not least in the changing world of medical sciences that the revolution in genomics and proteomics will bring. Advances in biological, medical and life sciences and especially those relating to the application of stem cells, pharmacogenomics and bioinformatics has, necessarily, raised entirely new issues in pharmaceutical ethics.

This book is a timely collation of the current state of wisdom in this important field which will be of relevance not only to those who research for future treatment and therapies but those whose role it is to deliver them to the benefit of the patients in the context of the societies in which they live.

Professor Trevor Jones
BPharm, Phd, Hon DSc,
FPS, CChem, FRSC,
FKC, MCPP, Hon FFPM

1

The Basis of Ethics

JON MERRILLS

Parkdale House, Nottingham, UK

Let's start by getting some terms clear:

- Ethics is the systematic study of what is right and good with respect to conduct and character (1).

There are several other definitions and explanations of pharmaceutical ethics which can be used:

- The beliefs and behaviours to which members of the profession subscribe (2).
- A critical evaluation of assumptions and arguments (3).
- A discussion about what ought to be done or ought not to be done—a discussion about normative behaviour in the context of issues raised in this book.

Ethics is concerned not only with making appropriate decisions about what we ought to do, but also with justifying those decisions.

An **ethical dilemma** exists where the answer to a particular situation is not clear, or where there is a choice of answers. The fact that there may be more than one solution to a problem is sometimes difficult for scientists to deal with. Scientists have been taught the scientific method, and the certainty of scientific laws. It is, though, the very stuff of law and philosophy. To quote a US writer: "An ethical dilemma occurs when there is a conflict of moral values, creating a situation in which there is no clear right or wrong answer or in which there may be more than one correct solution" (4).

Pharmaceutical Ethics. Edited by S. Salek and A. Edgar.

Ethics asks the question: "What should I do?" The process of answering the question may involve the examination of moral duty (5).

All members of the healthcare professions share some common values and principles concerning their duties to patients and their views of the purpose of their individual professions. What we value guides our actions, our judgements, and our attitude to certain situations. Values are what we believe.

What professionals value as professionals is codified or written up in the various codes of ethics, of which perhaps the best known to the public is the Hippocratic Oath of doctors (Table 1.1). There are two main elements in the Hippocratic Oath:

1. Inward-looking rules about respecting teachers, colleagues, etc.
2. Generalized rules to care for the patient, which can be criticized as being little more than definitions of a doctor.

There are a number of modern versions of the Hippocratic Oath, which serve to indicate the responsibilities of doctors to their patients. Mostly these are found within the statements of the World Medical Association.

Table 1.1   The Hippocratic Oath

I SWEAR by Apollo the physician and Aesculapius, and Health, and All-heal, and all the gods and goddesses, that, according to my ability and judgment, I will keep this Oath and this stipulation—to reckon him who taught me this Art equally dear to me as my parents, to share my substance with him, and relieve his necessities if required; to look upon his offspring in the same footing as my own brothers, and to teach them this art, if they shall wish to learn it, without fee or stipulation; and that by precept, lecture, and every other mode of instruction, I will impart a knowledge of the Art to my own sons, and those of my teachers, and to disciples bound by a stipulation and oath according to the law of medicine, but to none others. I will follow that system of regimen which, according to my ability and judgment, I consider for the benefit of my patients, and abstain from whatever is deleterious and mischievous. I will give no deadly medicine to any one if asked, nor suggest any such counsel; and in like manner I will not give to a woman a pessary to produce abortion. With purity and with holiness I will pass my life and practice my Art. I will not cut persons labouring under the stone, but will leave this to be done by men who are practitioners of this work. Into whatever houses I enter, I will go into them for the benefit of the sick, and will abstain from every voluntary act of mischief and corruption; and, further, from the seduction of females or males, of freemen and slaves. Whatever, in connection with my professional service, or not in connection with it, I see or hear, in the life of men, which ought not to be spoken of abroad, I will not divulge, as reckoning that all such should be kept secret. While I continue to keep this Oath unviolated, may it be granted to me to enjoy life and the practice of the art, respected by all men, in all times. But should I trespass and violate this Oath, may the reverse be my lot.

Source: From Harvard Classics Vol. 38, Copyright 1910 by P.F. Collier and Son. This text was placed in the public domain, June 1993.

Declaration of Geneva

The Declaration of Geneva, written in 1948 and revised in 1968 and again in 1983, is a modern version of the Hippocratic Oath (Table 1.2). Its main principles, as applied to doctors, are:

- to make the health of my patient my first consideration;
- to consecrate my life to the service of humanity;
- to respect my patients' secrets even after death;
- to prevent considerations of religion, nationality, race, party politics or social standing intervening between my duty and my patient;
- to maintain utmost respect for human life;
- not to use medical knowledge contrary to the laws of humanity.

The International Code of Medical Ethics 1949 (revised 1968)

Duties of doctors in general:

- A doctor must always maintain the highest standards of professional conduct.
- A doctor must practise his profession uninfluenced by motives of profit.

Other ethical statements include the following.

Table 1.2   The Declaration of Geneva

At the time of being admitted as a member of the Medical Profession I solemnly pledge myself to consecrate my life to the service of humanity.
I will give to my teachers the respect and gratitude which is their due.
I will practise my profession with conscience and dignity.
The health of my patient will be my first consideration.
I will respect the secrets which are confided in me.
I will maintain by all the means in my power the honour and the noble traditions of the medical profession.
My colleagues will be my brothers.
I will not permit considerations of religion, nationality, race, party politics or social standing to intervene between my duty and my patient.
I will maintain the utmost respect for human life from the time of conception: even under threat, I will not use my medical knowledge contrary to the laws of humanity.
I make these promises solemnly, freely and upon my honour.

Declaration of Helsinki 1964 (revised 1975 and 1983)

Following the 1947 Nuremberg Trials of Nazi war criminals, informed consent has applied to medical experimentation, according to the code now expressed in the Declaration of Helsinki:

- In any research the interests of subject must always prevail over interests of science and society.

Pharmacy Oaths

Graduates of some US pharmacy colleges still take an oath to serve the patient. One version is prepared by the American Association of Colleges of Pharmacy (Table 1.3). Dutch and French pharmacists also take an oath at the end of their university studies. As far as I know this is not done by English pharmacy graduates.

The oaths I have seen are similar to the Hippocratic Oath, and its modern versions.

A Pharmacy Code from a Medical Code?

It is interesting to compare the medical codes with what might be put into a pharmacy code. In fact they are very similar, since to an extent they deal in generalities, and all members of the healthcare professions share some common values and principles concerning their duties to patients and their views of the purpose of their individual professions. I would like

Table 1.3   US Pharmacy Oath: prepared by the American Association of Colleges of Pharmacy

---

At this time, I vow to devote my professional life to the service of all mankind through the profession of pharmacy.

I will consider the welfare of humanity and relief of human suffering my primary concerns.

I will apply my knowledge, experience and skills to the best of my ability to assure optimal drug therapy outcomes for the patients I serve.

I will keep abreast of developments and maintain professional competency in my profession of pharmacy.

I will maintain the highest principles of moral, ethical and legal conduct.

I will embrace and advocate change in the profession of pharmacy that improves patient care.

I take these vows voluntarily with the full realization of the responsibility with which I am entrusted by the public.

Source: Reproduced with permission of the American Association of Colleges of Pharmacy.

you to consider how, with but the slightest change, these medical codes could apply to pharmacy.

Consider an adaptation of the Declaration of Geneva: the only change needed is in the last principle:

- not to use *pharmaceutical* knowledge contrary to the laws of humanity.

This would give a Pharmacy Code reading as follows:

> At the time of being admitted as a member of the Pharmacy Profession I solemnly pledge myself to consecrate my life to the service of humanity.
> I will give to my teachers the respect and gratitude which is their due.
> I will practise my profession with conscience and dignity.
> The health of my patient will be my first consideration.
> I will respect the secrets which are confided in me.
> I will maintain by all the means in my power the honour and the noble traditions of the pharmacy profession.
> My colleagues will be my brothers.
> I will not permit considerations of religion, nationality, race, party politics or social standing to intervene between my duty and my patient.
> I will maintain the utmost respect for human life from the time of conception: even under threat I will not use my pharmaceutical knowledge contrary to the laws of humanity.
> I make these promises solemnly, freely and upon my honour.

Pharmacy Codes of Ethics

However, there have been a number of codes of ethics devised specifically for pharmacists:

- The first code of ethics of the American Pharmaceutical Association was published in 1852. It has been periodically updated since, with the latest revision dating from 1994.
- The first code of ethics of the Royal Pharmaceutical Society of Great Britain was published in 1944, after some years of discussion. Revised versions were produced at irregular intervals, in 1953, 1964, 1970 and 1984, and a new version is currently in preparation.
- The International Pharmaceutical Federation (FIP) issued a Code of Ethics for Pharmacy in 1997 which is intended to serve as a model for all the pharmacy organizations of the world. This Code contains nine principles supplemented by more detailed and explanatory obligations (Table 1.4).

Table 1.4   Principles in the code of ethics for pharmacists issued by the
International Pharmaceutical Federation in 1997

1. The pharmacist's prime responsibility is the good of the individual.
2. The pharmacist shows the same dedication to all.
3. The pharmacist respects the individual's right to freedom of choice of treatment.
4. The pharmacist respects and safeguards the individual's right to confidentiality.
5. The pharmacist co-operates with colleagues and other professionals and respects their values and abilities.
6. The pharmacist acts with honesty and integrity in professional relationships.
7. The pharmacist serves the needs of the individual, the community and society.
8. The pharmacist maintains and develops professional knowledge and skills.
9. The pharmacist ensures continuity of care in the event of labour disputes, pharmacy closure or conflict with personal moral beliefs.

Source: Reproduced with permission of the International Pharmaceutical Federation.

Why should we follow such declarations? Some countries include the professions' codes of practice in their laws, and the law should be obeyed. British pharmacists can argue that the only code of interest to them is the RPSGB Code. This is because all pharmacists practising in Great Britain are required to belong to the RPSGB and they are accustomed to following its pronouncements on practice matters. It forms a background against which actions of the pharmacist may be judged. In the UK a breach of the Code may constitute "professional misconduct" and lead to disciplinary action by the Statutory Committee. However, the RPSGB Code has no legal force, is not referred to in NHS legislation, and may be deviated from for good reason.

Thus the question is raised as to the basis of the authority of the codes. Is it just a legal one? What happens if law and ethics or morals differ? Which should be obeyed? Professor Hart, a lawyer, gives an example (6). A woman denounced her husband to the authorities for making insulting remarks about the country's ruler. Such insults were illegal under the written law. He was imprisoned. Some time later, when the government had changed, the woman was prosecuted under an earlier written law "for illegally depriving her husband of his freedom". She argued that as he had been imprisoned in accordance with the law of the time, there was no illegality. The court held that the later law, under which the husband was imprisoned, was so contrary to justice that it was not law. There is a suggestion here that written rules, whether laws or codes of ethics, do not stand totally alone and are justified by something. They are based on the "laws of humanity" which, depending on your personal point of view, justify right or wrong according to either "duty" or "consequence".

According to the first viewpoint we behave as we do out of duty. This group of theories is called "Deontological", derived from "deon", the Greek word for "duty". We obey the rules because we are under a duty to obey them, usually because the demand is a demand of the god, usually handed down to the people through a prophet—as with the Jewish view that Moses was given ten commandments, or in Islam through the words of the prophet Muhammad as recorded in the Koran.

Deontologists may also base the argument on the "law of nature"—a view that basic moral laws just exist, in the same way as the law of gravity.

The second major line of thinking—that of the "Consequentialists"— states that right or wrong depends upon the nature of the consequences of the action. We should look at what follows from our actions, what our actions cause. The great exponent of this thinking was Jeremy Bentham, who put forward Utilitarianism—"the greatest happiness of the greatest number".

Utilitarianism has a number of problems (7):

- what is happiness?
- how do we know when it is greatest?
- greatest number of who or what?

It is difficult for an individual to work out how to use resources to achieve utility, but as John Stuart Mill (8) pointed out in 1863, we can be guided by "rules of life", moral rules which contain the collected wisdom of mankind. Any version of Utilitarianism must be supplemented by ideas of justice or fairness.

The notion of "Utilitarianism" underlies both ethics and economics. There is a fundamental tenet of economics that resource allocation should be aimed at maximizing the benefits to society from the resources available. That is, resources should be used in the most efficient way possible.

Kant

A non-religious Deontological approach is that of Immanuel Kant, who developed the concept of a "supreme moral law" which binds all rational beings. Rational beings (excluding animals) possess an absolute moral value, they are "ends in themselves" and recognize themselves and other rational beings as such: "Act so that you treat humanity, whether in your own person or that of another, always as an end and never as a means only" (9).

This may be put (and is by many philosophers) that it is wrong to force another to do anything against his will. Nozick (10) states "Individuals are ends and not merely means; they may not be sacrificed or used for the achieving of other ends without their consent". This begins to suggest that there are somehow "rights" which people have and which cannot be taken from them.

Rights are justified claims that require action or restraint from others—
that is, they impose positive or negative duties on others. There are many
categories of rights:

- legal rights—given by law, defined, e.g. right to free schooling in UK;
- institutional rights—given by an institution to its members, e.g. right to
  use library in club;
- special moral rights (11)—e.g. rights set out in a contract agreement or
  relationship, for example to be repaid a debt, or the right of a child to
  support by a parent;
- moral or natural rights—unlike others cannot be withdrawn, although
  entitlement to access them may be proscribed by law, e.g. if right to life
  then this can be withdrawn by a court.

Libertarians refer to the "equal right of all men to be free" (12). Today we
recognize that our patient has rights.

Declaration of Lisbon 1981

This is of interest because it is concerned with rights of patients. That makes
it of particular interest to those healthcare professionals who seek to practise
according to the fledgling tenets of "pharmaceutical care", which clarifies
the relationship and responsibility to the patient:

- to choose a doctor freely;
- to be cared for by a doctor whose clinical and ethical judgements are free
  from outside interference;
- to accept or refuse treatment after receiving adequate information;
- to have his or her confidences respected;
- to die in dignity;
- to receive or decline spiritual and moral comfort including the help of a
  minister of an appropriate religion.

I referred at the beginning to a moral dilemma—the problem we have of
deciding what to do. One way of putting the issues of a moral dilemma is to
ask "is it right?" Another way is to ask "is it just?" The same problem arises
with Utilitarianism. What exactly do we mean by "just" or "fair"?

Theories of Justice

Many are ultimately based upon the ideas of the ancient Greek philosopher
Aristotle. He produced a formal theory of justice—"equals should be

treated equally and unequals should be treated unequally in proportion to the relevant inequalities". This distinguishes between two meanings of "justice"—that of overall good, and that of equality of treatment, which must be understood as meaning fair, proportionate treatment.

Probably the most influential theory of recent years is that developed by John Rawls in his book *A Theory of Justice* (13). Rawls discusses how a system of law, designed to achieve justice, might develop. Rawls envisages that self-interested, but rational individuals, who are unaware of their place in society, will choose the rules to govern their society. He argues that the rules thus chosen will be just rules. This justice results from the fact that those making the rules operate behind a "veil of ignorance" which renders them impartial. They therefore choose a system whose first principle is that people should have the maximum liberty compatible with the same degree of liberty for everyone. The second principle is that deliberate inequalities are unjust unless they work to the advantage of the least well off.

A rival, and very different, theory is that of Robert Nozick. It is expounded in his book *Anarchy, State and Utopia* (14). Central to Nozick's approach are two "rights":

- the right to life;
- the right to have possessions.

Nozick believes that no-one, including government, is entitled to take away anyone's possessions if they were gained without violating any rights of other people.

Marxist theories of justice, currently out of favour, are summed up by the phrase "to each according to his need, from each according to his ability" (15).

Relationship with Legal Requirements or Duties

Pharmaceutical ethics is not just the exercise of formulating a code of conduct, nor is it simply a sociological study of the rules under which the profession operates. Its ultimate purpose is to construct and defend a code of practice.

Ethics are internal to the profession, accepted by the profession, to establish and maintain it as an honourable profession. We are also expected to follow the laws of humanity. It is when we examine this area that we find the greatest difficulty in answering difficult questions about policy—because we may well find conflicts between the codes of our profession, and the requirements of the state/law/population generally.

Sometimes the existence of a strong code of ethics is seen by a Totalitarian regime as a barrier to its own total control. Consequently the regime must either alter or remove the perceived barrier. In 1917, following the Russian revolution, the Hippocratic Oath was suspended in Russia. It reappeared in a revised version in 1971. The revised version had considerable similarities with the Hippocratic Oath, in that it contained sections on the care of patients, the protection of confidentiality and the need to update and improve knowledge (16). It also contained a new clause: "To conduct all my actions according to the principles of the Communist morale, to always keep in mind the high calling of the Soviet physicians and the high responsibility I have to my people and the Soviet government". With the political changes in the former Soviet Union the Hippocratic Oath is being resurrected. I leave you to consider whether there might be conflict between the duty of a doctor and the duty to follow the Communist morale.

Others have pointed to such conflicts arising in a clearly democratic society such as the United States. In Illinois, for example, where the death penalty is enforced, death following lethal injection at state-ordered executions must be pronounced by a doctor. The state law violates the ethical precepts of the doctor. The state gives those doctors who participate immunity from professional disciplinary action. The state also suspends the law in relation to professional registration, which requires adherence to the ethics of the profession. It is this area which is of great fascination to me as a lawyer and a pharmacist. This is the area where law, ethics and pharmacy meet.

Recent Changes of Significance—Shift of Ethical Focus: An Example

The development of the concept of "pharmaceutical care" as the main statement of the purpose of the profession/aim of the profession/framework around which the role of the profession is articulated has eventually to be reflected in a changed ethics code. The duties and responsibilities of pharmacists are always related to the role which they play in society—whether that is as the mixers of medicines or as the experts in the use of medicines.

If the ultimate duty or responsibility of pharmacists is to contribute to the improvement in health of the patient by ensuring that the patient receives safe and effective pharmaceutical therapy, this means that the relationship with the patient is of higher importance than any other relationship. In other words, the patient comes first.

Pharmaceutical care challenges pharmacists to deliver the outcomes despite barriers, e.g. of professional views.

There will be more problems to be resolved as pharmacists, and other health professionals, cross some of the territorial boundaries which each healthcare profession currently sees as defining and delineating their individual roles. The simultaneous development of "patient-focused care" complicates this change. In "patient-focused care" teams of health professionals, from all the relevant disciplines, work in an integrated way to care for the patient. The individual members do not have sharply defined roles in relation to care functions, but are broadly interchangeable. They teach each other the skills which are needed to look after the patient. Thus a pharmacist may write up the script, or change the dressing, if that pharmacist is there at the appropriate time.

Pharmaceutical care will inevitably lead to conflicts—ethical dilemmas— when the duty to the patient cannot be met without jeopardizing some other important duty, e.g. to obey the law.

As the pharmacist pays more attention to the patient, as he becomes more patient-oriented, in order to improve that patient's quality of life, the responsibilities of Pharmaceutical Care expand. This is important because the pharmacist is more able to, and is expected to, intervene on behalf of the patient. This more personal relationship—as displayed by the use of the term "patient" rather than "customer"—brings with it more complex ethical dilemmas.

CONCLUSION

All healthcare professionals have to balance the needs of the individual patient against the needs of all their patients. An example would be the practice of "defensive medicine", where the fear of being sued for not doing a possibly unnecessary procedure is greater than the need of the patient to be invaded.

Where codes of ethics guarantee the independence of the healthcare professional involved, e.g. where the codes say that there should be no restriction on the right of a doctor to prescribe any treatment deemed necessary, there will automatically be a conflict with an economic perspective.

Where the codes speak of benevolence, some critics argue that they may lead to paternalism. For example, while most people are presumed to speak the truth, doctors decide what a patient needs to know for their own good. In many cultures bad news is never given to the patient, who is thereby deprived of autonomy in relation to decisions.

Indeed in the past some commentators, for example Professor Williams (17), have blamed "the dictates of medical ethics" for slowing the drive for greater efficiency in healthcare provision.

Continues

Continued

The notion of "Utilitarianism" also underlies both ethics and economics. There is a fundamental tenet of economics that resource allocation should be aimed at maximizing the benefits to society from the resources available. That is, resources should be used in the most efficient way possible.

In our world there is not enough money to go round. Treatments are rationed by money, whether that of the state or that of the individual. Decisions on resource allocation have to be made. The conflict between professional ethics and economics is there. What matters for patients are beneficence, non-maleficence and autonomy. What matters for society is an equitable distribution of resources.

Fortunately commentators such as Professor Raanan Gillon believe that in practice doctors are able to balance ethics and economics. Let us hope that other healthcare professionals and the pharma industry are able to do that as well.

REFERENCES

1. Weinstein B. *Am Pharm* 1993; **Sept**: 48.
2. *Philosophy and Practice of Medical Ethics*. BMA, 1988.
3. Raphael D. *Moral Philosophy*, 1981.
4. *Am Pharm* 1993; **Apr**.
5. Beauchamp TL and Childress JF. *Principles of Biomedical Ethics*, 1989.
6. Hart HLA. Positivism and the separation of law and morals. In *The Philosophy of Law*, Dworkin (ed), 1977.
7. Warnock M (ed). *Utilitarianism*, 1962.
8. Mill JS. *Utilitarianism*. Fontana, 1962.
9. Kant I. *Foundations of the Metaphysics of Morals*. CUP, 1991.
10. Nozick R. *Anarchy, State & Utopia*, 1974.
11. Gillon R. *Philosophical Medical Ethics*, 1986.
12. Hart HLA. In *Human Rights*, Melden (ed), 1970.
13. Rawls J. *A Theory of Justice*, 1976.
14. Nozick R. *Anarchy, State and Utopia*, 1974.
15. Marx K, Engels F. Manifesto of the Communist Party.
16. Presidium of the Highest Soviet of the USSR—The Oath of Soviet Physicians 1971. *JAMA* 1995; **273** (20).
17. Williams A. *Medical Ethics, Health Service Efficiency and Clinical Freedom*, 1985.

2

Principles of Ethics Focusing on the Patient

ANDREW EDGAR
Centre for Applied Ethics, Philosophy Section,
University of Wales, Cardiff, UK

This chapter will address two core questions with respect to the relationship of ethics to pharmaceutical research and clinical practice: 1. What is the purpose of teaching ethics? 2. Why are the patient's understanding of, and attitude towards, research and clinical practice important from a moral perspective?

The first question entails that we ask how an awareness of ethics might change the understanding that researchers and clinicians have of their work, and how that awareness might influence everyday working practices. It also leads to an initial account of ethics as an awareness of practice that makes it more (not less) problematic. This is because professional and scientific practice can be ethical only by respecting the different viewpoints and understandings of others. This provides the context for asking the second question.

The second question entails that we recognize that patients and the lay public may have a different understanding of the nature, purpose and priorities of research and clinical practice than that held by the medical or pharmaceutical profession. If this assertion is plausible, then one must inquire into the precise consequences that recognition of the patient's perspective has for the scientist or professional. The assessment of consequences in turn depends upon asking whether or not the patient's perspective has any worth or value. (Bluntly, one must ask whether patients and the public are merely ill-informed or confused, or do they have a distinctive and important understanding of disease, health and medicine?)

Pharmaceutical Ethics. Edited by S. Salek and A. Edgar.

This is an ethical question, for it is to ask if the views of patients and the public should be taken seriously, and if so, how the clinician and researcher should respond to them and allow them to influence professional practice and decision-making. Equally, it is to recognize that the medical professional may have an obligation to educate and inform patients and the public, in order to challenge and change mistaken understandings and opinions.

THE PURPOSE OF ETHICS

The question of exactly what ethics is—the problem of defining "ethics"—is a surprisingly difficult one to resolve with any precision. Crudely, ethics concerns the way in which human beings behave, and more specifically, the way in which we behave towards each other. It concerns what is good for humans, and as such entails that we respect human fulfilment, happiness and worth. To make a moral decision is therefore to make a decision that takes due account of the interests, goals and well-being of other human beings.

In order to examine the implications and uses that ethical teaching might have for professional practice, we look briefly at two accounts (or models) of ethics and ethical decision-making. On the first account, ethics may be encapsulated in a set of more or less abstract rules (or principles) that may then be used to guide the practitioner, specifically in resolving the moral dilemmas that he or she encounters. Such dilemmas might be characterized in terms of a conflict between the interests of the people involved in the situation. The moral dilemma is resolved, as best it might be, by applying a general principle (or set of such principles) to the situation.

The "principlist" approach, as it is known, would proceed as follows. Four general principles are proposed to guide moral practice: non-maleficence (the doctor should do no unnecessary harm); beneficence (the doctor should do good); autonomy (the doctor should respect the autonomy of the patient); justice (the doctor should treat patients equitably and fairly, respecting relevant similarities and differences between them, when determining the treatment that they should receive). Faced with a moral dilemma, the medical professional uses these principles to guide his or her reflection as to the most appropriate course of action. A variation on this approach would be the recognition of a few core ethical ideas or concepts that guide action. These would include those of "informed consent" and "confidentiality", both of which have their grounding in the principle of respect for patient autonomy.

Such an approach is extremely important, and has proved of great value (not least in the development of medical ethics as a practical resource for medical professionals) (1–3). It is an excellent place from which to begin teaching and learning medical ethics. Its importance lies, especially, in the fact that it makes clear that ethical decision-making requires reasoning, rather than intuitive responses. An action is justified, not because it is merely felt to be right, but because it can be defended through an appeal to the principles. The principles themselves can be defended through a further level of reasoning (that serves to ground the principles in more general understandings of the nature of ethics, of the good life and of human nature). However, I want to express a number of reservations about principlism, or more properly, unreflective or habitual approaches to principlism. I want to suggest that while it may be a beginning to ethical teaching, it can never be the end, not least because it may prematurely cut short the process of ethical reasoning, and therefore should never be seen as an exhaustive account of ethics.

My first reservation is that the principlist approach, and indeed the related dependence on a few core moral ideas (such as informed consent), too readily assumes that moral dilemmas do have solutions, and that the principles are the largely unproblematic key to finding those solutions. An overly simplistic approach to the use of moral principles may lead to moral dilemmas being treated as being akin to technical problems. The appropriate application of a general principle (akin to the correct calculation of the force to be exerted by a lever) will resolve the problem (at least as well as it can be resolved). The practitioner would then no more need to reflect upon the justification of the principles used than would the engineer have to justify the theory of gravity. The principles would be merely accepted as encapsulating moral wisdom, much as the laws of Newtonian physics once encapsulated the knowledge of physics.

This reservation can be explicated by suggesting that principlism can be insensitive to the irresolvable tragedy of moral dilemmas. Something of the importance of this reservation may be illustrated as follows. Mortality rates are frequently used as an indication of the effectiveness and efficiency of hospitals. The introduction of mortal "league tables" might be given cautious approval by appeal to the four principles. The publication of this information respects autonomy, for it gives patients more information upon which to base their choices about health care. In addition, the effective use of scarce health care resources is at least a part of what is entailed in ensuring the just use of those resources. Finally, if death may readily be regarded as the most extreme harm that can befall a patient, then low mortality rates would indicate a hospital that is maximizing good (beneficence) and avoiding harm (non-maleficence).

The following example indicates the problematic nature of such an approach. If a hospital is to maintain low death rates, then the death of neonates is to be avoided. Yet certain medical conditions, such as encephalitis, entail that the death of the neonate is highly likely within hours or at most days of birth. To avoid this death, and thus to avoid the impact that such a death would have on mortality rates, if encephalitis is diagnosed through prenatal screening, then an abortion could be offered. The abortion would be a successful operation, in contrast to the undesirable death. This example is intended to throw into question exactly how undesirable death actually is. If the pregnancy is brought to term then, with a little cosmetic help, the parents can have a child to cuddle and photograph, and a child to mourn. Family and friends are likely to gather round in support of the bereaved couple. An abortion, in contrast, may lead to feelings of guilt and to social isolation.

wow

From this example it may be argued that the very nature of good and harm can be contested, and thus that it is too simplistic to assume that there is a single, overwhelming solution to a moral dilemma. It might rather be argued that different perspectives (such as that of doctor against that of patient) lead to different solutions, although, as the above example also suggests, there are few solutions that are not tinged with suffering and tragedy. It is perhaps necessary to note that while bringing the pregnancy to term may, morally, be the preferred action, the child still dies, and the death may well appear to be senseless to the parents. A principlist approach (or perhaps more properly, an unimaginative and too hasty application of principlism) may therefore overlook something that should be fundamental to medical ethics, and indeed to medicine itself: that medicine is ultimately about humanity's confrontation with its own mortality. One might add that a similar insensitivity characterizes biomedical models of health and illness (which is to say, those models that treat illness and disease merely as dysfunctions in a complex organism) (4). Medical ethics, at the very least, should resist such models, and should not therefore mimic them in its own pattern of reasoning.

My first reservation, that principlism may lead to too simplistic a view of the complexity, not simply of moral dilemmas but also of medical practice itself, is implicated with another reservation: that principlism is too readily associated with a legal approach to medical practice, and that the legal and the moral do not necessarily coincide. Ideas such as informed consent and confidentiality are readily (and quite properly) incorporated into the legal regulation of the medical professions. However, the practice of the doctor can then become that of avoiding legal prosecution (in a "defensive medicine" that avoids the threat of legal action by the patient, or ensures that actions have been taken to win any such legal action). Thus, the medical professional may be seen as avoiding moral condemnation by checking a questionable or troublesome decision against the four principles. While this is understandable, it is not necessarily moral (or at best, is an impoverished approach to morality, that seeks mere peace of mind rather than moral growth). As Jan Payne observes in this volume, what matters is not the word or name "informed consent", but rather the concept and thought that lies behind that name. Informed consent is not secured, morally, by the routine and unreflective request for a patient's signature on a consent form. The treatment of informed consent as little more than a formal gesture, which is to say as a legal prerequisite to treatment, divorces it from due consideration of the risks that the patient is likely to undergo, and thus the need to communicate, appropriately, with the patient, in order to ensure that he or she has indeed understood those risks, and that the consent given is genuinely unforced.

A third and final reservation may be noted. As an approach to problem-solving, principlism assumes that one recognizes a moral dilemma when it is encountered. However, it is being suggested here that the objective of ethics teaching might be understood less in terms of the solution of known and recognized problems than in the recognition of previously unknown problems. To some extent, principlism (and such related ideas as informed consent and confidentiality) do perform the role of making the medical professional more sensitive to the moral dimension of actions and choices. The principles serve to draw the doctor's attention to the complexities of balancing harms and goods, or respecting autonomy and treating patients equitably. Thus, for example, an explicit awareness of the relationship of beneficence and non-maleficence may alert the researcher to moral dimensions in clinical trials and statistical analysis. In accord with non-maleficence, the researcher may ask whether a randomized control trial should be ended as soon as unambiguous data are available as to the efficacy of a new pharmaceutical product (either to avoid further risk to those research subjects taking a new drug, or to avoid unnecessary harm, through lack of effective treatment, of those taking a placebo). Similarly, moral debates have been generated over the relative merits of Bayesian and classical statistics. Proponents of Bayesian statistics argue that clear results are generated more quickly, thereby reducing risks to research subjects. Thus, even the rarefied and seemingly objective world of statistical analysis can be revealed to have a moral dimension (5).

Despite the positive role that the principles can play, they still presuppose a certain conception of the moral dilemma, and perhaps more importantly a certain conception of the role of the actors within this dilemma. The historical origin of the principles is such that they are of particular relevance to medical practice as it developed after the Second World War, and perhaps more significantly, as it developed in the United States. As an ethics of research, principlism (along with such core ethical concepts as informed consent) grows out of the shadow of Nazism and the Nuremberg Trials. As a professional ethics, it responds to a shift in the relationship between doctor and patient: as patients became increasing well educated (with the post-war expansion of mass education and middle-class occupations), better organized (with the rise of pressure groups defending patients' interests) and better informed. In the United States, this perhaps also reflects the increasingly contractual nature of the relationship between patient and doctor (that in turn is reflected in the legalism of principlism).

Principlism still, however, tends to assume that there is a knowledgeable medical professional who is confronted by the moral dilemma. The dilemma is his or her responsibility. In contrast the patient, while given a certain amount of respect through the principle of autonomy, is assumed to be largely passive. The acquisition of moral knowledge (in the form of the principles) will complement the scientific and therapeutic knowledge that the medical professional already has. He or she will then be able to act on the patient's behalf. Professional paternalism may therefore be modified, as a more subtle account of the patient's interests is placed at the forefront of the decision-making process, but it is not entirely removed. Principlism merely makes clear the point that purely technical knowledge is insufficient for the modern doctor.

The fact that medical practice and medical research continues to develop (with new challenges posed by both technological developments within medicine, and perhaps more importantly by demographic, economic and cultural changes to the environment within which medicine is practised) not only entails that an unreflective principlist approach may be unable to cope with the complex and as yet unknown and unrecognized problems of the future. More importantly, principlism, by taking for granted a historically and culturally specific relationship between patient and doctor (or patient and researcher) may not be able to reflect upon the moral problems that are inherent in that very relationship. For example, if the relationship between doctor and patient is becoming increasingly impersonal and contractual, then an approach to ethics that takes contractualism for granted may be unable to ask whether or not this is a morally suitable model for the doctor–patient relationship. (It may indeed be suggested that principlism has had less influence in Western Europe than in the United States, because the relationship between the European doctor and his or her patient is less contractually and legally based.) An unreflective approach to principlism (which is to say, an approach that accepts the principles are given, without inquiring into the deeper reasoning and presuppositions that ground them) may, therefore, be unable to recognize the most fundamental moral problems that are hidden in its very assumptions.

I have therefore suggested that an unreflective principlism (or an approach to principlism that regards it as an exhaustive account of medical ethics, rather than as the beginning of a moral reflection and reasoning) can lead to an impoverished and mechanical view of what moral problems are, and so, paradoxically, can make the practitioner insensitive to moral problems (and most importantly to the unavoidably tragic nature of many moral decisions), simply because they do not fall readily within the terms of principlist thinking.

My alternative model of ethics entails an approach known as "discourse ethics" (6,7). In the principlist model, the individual practitioner appears to reflect, in isolation, on the moral dilemma with which he or she is confronted. It was suggested above that the principlist approach assumes that the moral responsibility is the practitioner's, and thus it may be added, it is the responsibility of the practitioner, alone, to work out the solution to the moral dilemma. Philosophy itself has long suffered from this solipsistic model of reasoning (at least since Descartes attempted to reconstruct human knowledge on certain foundations, through the pure thought experiment of doubting everything that could be doubted) (8). In contrast, a discourse ethics approach assumes that human beings are social creatures, and as such, the knowledge, ability and sensitivity of the individual is advanced through engagement with other individuals. Thus, ethical decision-making is seen to lie in the openness of the individual to the insights, challenges and experiences of others. Decisions are made, not through the rational reflection of one individual, but through debate and discussion by all who will be affected by the decision. It accepts that all decisions that are made are likely to be imperfect, and that they will be open to revision in the light of new experiences or arguments.

A discourse ethics approach assumes that a moral decision is well made when all people involved have been free to express any views that they have and to raise any problems or reservations about the decision (including their simple inability to understand what is going on). Not only may the particular interpretation and application of moral principles or concepts be challenged, but so may the ideas that ground those principles. A viewpoint can only be excluded from debate on the grounds that it is irrational or ill-informed. As such, discourse ethics demands a certain humility on the part of all participants to the discussion, for they must not only be willing to listen, seriously and attentively, to the views and arguments of others, but they must be willing to allow the most coherent and well-informed argument to prevail, and so they must be willing to abandon their own position if it is shown to be flawed.

In practice, such open debate occurs rarely. Free debate is an ideal. Discourse ethics is aware of this, but does not then see that it is necessary to abandon free debate as an ideal. Rather, by recognizing the difference between the real and the ideal, the moral philosopher distinguishes his or her own position and tasks from that of the practitioner and lay person. The task of resolving moral dilemmas (even if the resolution is provisional) falls on the people involved. It is their problem, and they will have the experience and commitment necessary to deal with the problem, and will have to bear the burden of failure. The task of the moral philosopher, in contrast, is to examine the manner in which that resolution is brought about, and to identify where it has fallen short of the ideal, and why, and thus to provide participants with the intellectual resources necessary to improve real debate. Two forms of imperfection may be anticipated. On the one hand, the participants may lack the resources to resolve the debate to everyone's satisfaction. They may lack relevant scientific knowledge (for example, of the physical or psychological effects of a drug or treatment), or the ability to communicate that knowledge effectively. They may even lack the imagination or sensitivity to recognize a problem as a moral problem. On the other hand, certain people may be excluded from the debate, so that their views are not heard or are ignored. This exclusion can take many forms, and the identification and explanation of exclusion is the central concern of discourse ethics. Thus, it has been suggested above that a paternalistic model of medicine (where "doctor knows best") may serve to exclude patients and lay people from the decision-making process. Crucially, this is unacceptable if it is based upon an unconsidered view of medical practice (or upon mere prejudices about the patient), and is enforced by the medical profession exercising its greater power simply to silence or ignore the voice of the patient. Inequalities of power are a crucial factor in distorting communication. A more problematic example occurs when the exclusion is based on the judgement of the irrelevance or incoherence of a person's views and opinions.

THE PATIENT'S PERSPECTIVE

If there is any plausibility in the above account of discourse ethics, then the incorporation of the patient's views and values into the moral decision-making process is essential. Ideally, there should be open and equal discussion between the patient and the medical professionals in the resolution of any problem (or indeed in the determination of the course of a treatment). Such discussion would allow the patient to express his or her goals and values, and thus allow, for example, the doctor to recognize that the profession's understanding of successful treatment need not necessarily coincide with the patient's conception. However, if practice falls short of any such ideal, then the core issue of ethical decision-making becomes that of negotiating, managing and learning from imperfections.

The medical patient, and indeed the lay participant in research, is vulnerable. The imperfection of any dialogue between doctor and patient lies precisely in this vulnerability. The patient, because he or she is a patient, is suffering some physical or mental incompetence. Pain, fear, confusion and frustration may all serve to inhibit the patient's ability to make decisions (even about what is in his or her own best interest), or to engage in rational and well-informed discussion with a doctor or nurse. Given the incapacity of the patient, it is tempting for the doctor to assume that he or she does indeed know best, and thus to take responsibility for the patient. Similarly, it is all too easy to consider views and values that diverge from those of the doctor or the medical profession to be a result of the imbalances brought on by the illness, rather than the result of mature reflection by an autonomous patient. A benign paternalism might then be adopted, for however attractive the ideal of open communication and decision-making might be, it is impracticable in most medical circumstances (and reverting to principlism, the most appropriate way to respect patient autonomy would be to bring about a cure as quickly as possible, thereby restoring that autonomy).

Further, regardless of the patient's physical or mental vulnerability, the doctor (or medical researcher) will hold more power than the patient, because the doctor is better educated (at least about the disease or injury from which the patient is suffering), and is likely to have greater institutional and cultural power. The doctor is in what, to him or her, are familiar surroundings, accompanied and supported by colleagues. In addition, the doctor may still be a figure who is traditionally respected. The ideas of informed consent and confidentiality do much to recognize the vulnerability and powerlessness of the patient, and to give protection.

Despite its apparent emphasis on the ideal of equal and open discussion, the approach to ethics that I have suggested does take the problems of vulnerability, power and paternalism seriously, precisely because it highlights the divergence of the real from the ideal, and as such recognizes that there is no easy solution to real problems. The ideal of open communication may be impracticable, but its importance as an ideal is that it draws attention to practical imperfections (thus making us aware of moral problems where they might otherwise go unnoticed), and continues to demand that some approximation to the ideal is sought. Thus, for example, despite their importance, the demand for informed consent and confidentiality do not resolve problems, and if used unthinkingly, without due respect for the problems of communicating with the patient, may be mere stop-gaps that lead to continuing abuse.

The problem of the patient's perspective is therefore a problem of communication between doctor and patient (as John Lilja reflects upon elsewhere in this volume), and that in turn rests upon the more profound and taxing problem of recognizing when the patient is the best judge of his or her own interests, and so when the patient's views should have precedence over the doctor's, and conversely when the doctor's paternalism is in fact justified. The complexities of this point may be illustrated.

First, one might consider the problem of telling the patient the truth about his or her illness. A personal experience may illustrate this point. On a recent visit to Moldavia, I spoke to oncologists about medical ethics. In the course of conversation, it turned out that these doctors did not tell their patients that they had cancer, and positively forbade relatives from informing the patients. This apparent abuse of the informed consent was justified by the observation that, in Moldavia, people assumed that cancer was a terminal disease, beyond effective treatment. The very belief that one had cancer might there contribute to one's poor prognosis.

Superficially, the ideal of open communication would suggest that the doctor has an obligation to inform the patient. An ideal patient would want to know the truth of his or her condition, and would cooperate with the doctor in its treatment or management. Yet the patient, almost by definition, is not ideal. The physically or psychologically weakened patient may be even less capable of handling news of his or her own mortality than the rest of us. Further, as the experience of Moldavia emphasizes, in a culture that does not talk of or acknowledge death or is ill-informed about a particular disease, the problem becomes more acute, as the doctor may lack the cultural resources that would allow the patient to make sense of the illness. Notably, the oncologists in Moldavia thought that they might have a moral obligation to publicize successful cancer treatment as widely as possible. The decision to inform or not to inform the patient is therefore fraught with risk. Although, again, the more the doctor recognizes his or her own incompetence in judging a patient and in talking to the patient, the more cautiously the decision will be made. This is turn entails making the decision in consultation with others, be they other professionals or the patient's relatives and friends.

Second, we may return to the problem of acquiring a patient's informed consent. Much empirical and theoretical work has already been carried out to demonstrate the problems inherent in gaining truly informed consent from a patient. The complex medical language of the doctor or researcher has to be translated into terms that the patient will understand, and has to be given in small enough packages for the patient to absorb. It may need to be repeated or reinforced in subsequent discussions. Such observations, which are extremely important, serve to emphasize, again, the patient's incompetence. The patient, naturally enough, is unable to understand the complex technical information that grounds the doctor's decision to prescribe a particular treatment. However, one might equally turn the issue about, and inquire into the doctor's competence in understanding a patient.

The movement towards increased use of quality of life measures, both in allocating health care resources and in assessing the efficacy of medical interventions, has great potential in allowing the values and views of the patient to be heard in medical decision-making. The more sophisticated quality of life measures currently being used (such as the Sickness Impact

Profile, SF-36 and SEIQoL) are constructed through consultation with lay people, in order to establish how both health and illness should be described if they are to be relevant to the experience of lay people. The parameters of health (and their description) are derived from public surveys. In addition, the values or weights given to the various health states so described are again derived through public consultation. At the very least, a quality of life measure therefore provides a picture of lay views and attitudes towards health and illness that may pose a challenge to the medical professional. For example, the routine inclusion of social and emotional aspects in quality of life measures reminds the medical professional that illness is more than a mere dysfunction in a biological organism.

The increasing popularity of homeopathic medicine, throughout the United States and Europe, throws further light on the ethical relationship between patients and the medical profession. From the scientific perspective of the doctor or pharmacist, the use of homeopathic medicines is irrational. The consumption of homeopathic medicine is grounded in a lack of adequate scientific education, and a confused idea of benign "natural" products. While this may appear to justify the exclusion of the proponents of alternative or complementary medicines from the debate over health care, and thus to justify medical paternalism through an appeal to good science, this would be too hasty a conclusion. The use of alternative medicine is not simply grounded in ignorance, but also reflects the failure of orthodox medicine to meet the needs and expectations of patients and the public. [The incidence of adverse drug reactions, for example, suggests that orthodox medicine has no grounds for complacency (9).] The use of homeopathic medicine is thus symptomatic of a wide range of failings on the part of medicine and pharmacy. In part, such failings are failures of communication (e.g. to communicate the real benefits and risks of pharmaceuticals, and the limits as well as the benefits of medical technology). But such failings are also indicative of the way in which orthodox medicine deals with patients. Homeopathic medicine may appear to give the patient greater autonomy and control over his or her treatment, and in addition a treatment that responds to the whole person, rather than to a mere biological organism. Homeopathic medicine may therefore be more sensitive to the vulnerability of the patient than is orthodox medicine. (The use of homeopathic medicine may therefore send a very similar message to orthodox medical practice to that offered by the quality of life movement.) To the lay person, homeopathic medicine may appear to be closer to an ideal of open communication between equals than is orthodox medicine.

Finally, while much medical ethics focuses on potential conflicts between the doctor and patient, one may also usefully inquire critically into the reasons why a patient agrees with a doctor. Ideally, of course, agreement occurs because the doctor is acting in the best interests of the patient, and the patient recognizes that beneficent paternalism for what it is. Yet, if the ideal of open and informed communication is to be questioned elsewhere, then it should also be questioned here, when agreement occurs. Agreement itself may rest in the vulnerability and powerlessness of the patient. The patient may concur with the doctor because he or she is in awe of the doctor's power and status. It may not even occur to the patient to question or challenge the doctor.

CONCLUSION

In conclusion, I should return briefly to the two questions with which I began this chapter: 1. What is the purpose of teaching ethics? 2. Why are the patient's understanding of, and attitude towards, research and clinical practice important from a moral perspective? I have tried to suggest that the purpose of teaching ethics is to force the physician and the researcher to reflect upon their activities, and to take as little as is humanly possible for granted. This reflection, in answer to the second question, necessarily involves the patient, for it must take place as a real dialogue and not a monologue (or even as a dialogue between physicians alone). To bring the patient into the discussion, and thus to engage with the patient's perspective, involves taking account of someone who is vulnerable before the power of the medical profession. Such engagement therefore makes professional practice more difficult and more problematic. One cannot act like an engineer, simply applying the appropriate principles in order to calculate the best possible outcome, and nor, ethically, should one act with one eye on the possibility of legal proceedings. Instead, the power of the medical profession perhaps places upon it a responsibility to facilitate the patient's participation in discussion as a reasonable and well-informed disputant. The results will be imperfect. Critical debate does not end conclusively, but only temporarily and uncertainly, for typically one must act in some degree of ignorance of the consequences of one's actions, and even of the full motivations and reasons that have led to that particular course of action. Ultimately, to act ethically is not, necessarily, to act perfectly. It is rather to act upon careful consideration of the best information and opinion available, and if the act turns out badly, to act ethically is to acknowledge one's errors and learn from one's mistakes.

REFERENCES

1. Beauchamp TL, Childress JF. *Principles of Biomedical Ethics*, 4th edn. Oxford University Press: New York, 1994.
2. Gillon R. *Philosophical Medical Ethics*. John Wiley: Chichester, 1986.
3. Gillon R (ed). *Principles of Health Care Ethics*. John Wiley: Chichester, 1994.
4. Boorse C. Health as a theoretical concept. *Philos Sci* 1977; **44**: 542–73.
5. Hutton JL. The ethics of randomised controlled trials: A matter of statistical belief. *Health Care Anal* 1996; **4** (2): 95–102.
6. Habermas J. *Moral Consciousness and Communicative Action*. MIT Press: Cambridge, MA, 1990.
7. Benhabib S, Dallmayr F (eds). *The Communicative Ethics Controversy*. MIT Press: Cambridge, MA, 1990.
8. Sorell T. *Descartes*. Oxford University Press: Oxford, 1987.
9. Lazarou J, Pomeranz BH, Corey PN. Incidence of adverse drug reactions in hospitalized patients: A meta-analysis of prospective studies. *J Am Med Assoc* 1998; **279**: 1200–5.

3

Ethical Rationalism Applied to Pharmaceuticals

R.P. DESSING

Apotheek AAN ZEE, Noordwijk, The Netherlands

SUMMARY

To find ethical guidelines for pharmacy practice today seems rather complicated. Moral principles which are based on religion or on Western–Greek–
Jewish–Christian tradition are not self-evident any more. Today's society
asks for a rational approach to problems that result from conflicting interests of all kinds, including topics in health care. This chapter tries to develop
a reasoning that can be applied to the development and use of pharmaceuticals. General principles, based on accepted values in Western society such
as autonomy, democracy and solidarity, lead to guidelines for ethical behaviour. The chapter focuses on the aspects of cost control and pharmaceutical care. It concludes that protocols are important tools for everyday
practice. Pharmacists should focus more on negative outcomes of pharmacotherapy. Monitoring of patient care, identification and prevention of
possible adverse effects, medication surveillance, communication and information about proper use of medicines are priority items within our profession. A suggestion for a general code of ethics is proposed.

Keywords: Adverse effects; Autonomy; Cost control; Ethics; Euthanasia;
Human Genome Project; Medication surveillance; Pharmaceutical care;
Pharmacoeconomics; Pharmacovigilance; Pharmacy; Pharmacy profession;
Philosophy

Pharmaceutical Ethics. Edited by S. Salek and A. Edgar.
© 2002 John Wiley & Sons, Ltd.

INTRODUCTION

Many of us use the word ethics or the idea ethics whenever we are in a position to reflect on conflicting interests of individuals, groups or systems. In private, professional or in public life, choices, whether explicitly stated or not, have to be made on various occasions. The basis on which these choices are made is often created by traditional elements mixed with emotional and practical motives, rather than by a careful analysis of moral incentives in today's human behaviour.

This chapter tries to build up a rationality based on principles that have been generally respected and accepted in Western society for almost a century. It seeks to apply this to the practice of pharmacy and to related fields in health care.

MORAL PHILOSOPHY

As a first step, the nature of today's Western society, its organization and its individuals, is analysed in terms of belief, values and practical behaviour. Moral values and ethics do not seem to be dependent on metaphysical principles any more (1). Moral principles as symptoms of something that rises above culture and tradition seems to be something objective. But till now it has not been possible to prove that such supracultural principles have eternal validity (2). The only thing you could suggest was that, if there is a set of "universal" principles, these will manifest themselves in different ways in different places and at different times, depending on culture and tradition.

As an example, one could define the virtues defined by Aristotle as supracultural values (3). His basic presumption was that every art and inquiry, every action and choice was thought to aim at some "good". This "good" was meant as "good in itself". This "good" was connected with happiness. It was an activity of the soul in conformity with excellence, the best form of excellence. Moral excellence means that we must have knowledge and choices, and any action must proceed from a firm and unchangeable state. The best state is the intermediate between excess and deficit. It is a position equidistant from each of two extremes. Moral excellence is the consequence of a choice, determined by reason: the reason of a man of practical wisdom. Virtue was a mean between two vices. But one should accept that every culture explains and applies these virtues in its own way. We don't even know exactly how they were understood at the time and place of their conception.

A second important example of a philosopher who tried to formulate these "eternal values" was Kant. His construction of ethical principles is elegant and merely metaphysical in nature. He states that all moral concepts have their seat and origin in reason fully "a priori". They cannot be abstracted from any empirical knowledge. His main "universal principle", that "I should always act in such a way that my behaviour could be a universal law of nature", is disputable (4). An interesting point is that Kant claimed that we are not only bound by this law but can consider ourselves as authors of this law at the same time. Thus introducing the concept of autonomy. The concept of people being free human beings, free to think and free to act in matters of morality, but following the will as a law in itself in such a way that the "maxims" of your choice are also present as a universal law. The strong metaphysical aspects of this theory undermine its acceptance by today's society. But applications can still be recognized in many legislations, in the declaration of human rights (5) and in publications about ethics.

Analytical Philosophy: Ethics in the Third Millennium

If we accept that there is no set of universal and transculturally valid moral principles, then the local conception of what is a "good" life, a "happy" life, a "healthy" life and what is "quality" plays an important role. It implies that ethics should be observed through the windows of time and place. As a consequence, my view of ethics and the application of this to the pharmacy profession will be developed from values that we consider in our Western culture as fundamental.

An example of a value which can be considered as basic is the individual's autonomy. Autonomy can be defined as the individual's right or freedom to exist, to act, to think and to communicate (5). A definition of this principle will give important motivation to moral and ethical guidelines. Through this perception morality and ethics can be developed in a rational way. It implies that new moral principles can be introduced, after a careful analysis and a thorough debate with participation of the parties directly involved and with society. This point reveals a connection to the Greek philosophers: it was Aristotle who explained that ethics meant acting within and with society itself. Politics legislates as to what we are to do and what we are to abstain from. In other words, ethics was connected to politics, to the public life (6). It decided what should be good for man and for society in the end.

This approach demonstrates the limitations of the autonomy concept. We all agree that democratic rules should be respected, as they represent a synthesis or equilibrium between individual autonomy and man being part of society. The political basis for individual liberty was formulated by the French thinker Montesquieu. This principle can function on various levels. But in practice our society is organized as a state, and democracy organized on the system of "trias politica" is the current reality. This means the separation between the legislative, executive and judicial powers. Through the common interests of all individuals, democracy will result in a form of solidarity. It will not result in the *maximum* form of solidarity as proposed by Levinas (7), where only the OTHER is the leading principle. In this abstract and strictly philosophical approach, the choice between personal interest and the interest of the other human being will always be in the interest of the OTHER. It would be impossible to make any choice in personal life (8).

To summarize: our reasoning implies that ethics and morality are a result of a rationality, not of some supernatural objectivity.

The Practice of Pharmacy

If the individual's autonomy is an important leading principle in contemporary morality, all efforts of society should be mobilized to maintain this ability. Disease is one of the conditions that affects or at least threatens autonomy. At this point the connection between various health professions and this fundamental ethical principle is revealed. In medical practice and related pharmacy practice, the activities of professionals should be aimed at analysing where, how and to what degree the individual's autonomy is threatened or compromised. This could happen in any of the elements or fields which are covered by the foregoing definition: "freedom to exist, to think, to act and to communicate". The request of the patient to the health care provider will always relate to this principle. But to regard a person who is a "patient" as an autonomous human being is more complicated than it seems at first sight.

As an example, take autonomy as seen in terms of civil rights. Under law, a person has a democratic right to vote until the last second of his life and almost regardless of his mental or physical condition. In health care the mental and physical state will determine whether a part of the individual's right to decide is (perhaps unintentionally) taken away and transferred to some "professional". Later, I will refer to this in the framework of "informed consent", as part of this process. In practice, a patient with an illness or health problems will ask for help. This means in terms of life dynamics that a patient asks for assistance to inhibit possible worsening factors, to stabilize their personal health condition and if possible for a total restoration of autonomy.

If we apply these principles to the field of pharmacy, we can identify some guidelines needed for day-to-day problems in hospital and community practice. All solutions will be developed around the aforementioned theme and will have a similar approach: the proper assessment of the factors which threaten personal autonomy and which are therefore subject to inter-action between patient and health care professional. This will include a closer look at the techniques required to get proper access not only to the body but also to the "mind" of the patient in order to verify that both parties understand each other properly in respect of the personal health topic (9). I state explicitly "both parties" because autonomy is connected with every individual, including the health professional.

CASE 1: Autonomy and Solidarity in Health Care

Is it immoral to discuss cost in health care (10)? Is it unethical beha-viour to refuse treatment to a specific patient for financial reasons? Today it is clear that the costs of drug treatment are in competition with the costs of other fields of care: care for the elderly, care for the mentally ill, drug addicts, etc. This reveals fundamental and contro-versial interests, and it implies that ethical questions are at stake. As we pointed out before, the individual's autonomy is one of the leading principles and an important cornerstone for ethical behaviour. But at the same time we know that a compromise between this autonomy and general interests is necessary to avoid a climate of anarchy.

In daily life, these types of compromises are realized on many levels. To compromise in this respect is in fact an important result of our upbringing. On a larger scale, in society we know that total autonomy without a controlling system would result in the strongest individuals making the rules. A society would emerge where a large part of the population would be condemned to poverty and depen-dence, a society where many health provisions would not be accessi-ble for a significant part of the population. Such a picture is recognizable to some minority groups in various mega-cities in the (Western) world.

These limitations for individual behaviour and their political con-sequences were already recognized by the American philosopher Richard Rorty in his book *Contingency, Irony and Solidarity* (11). The idea that modern liberal societies are bound together by philosophical beliefs seems ludicrous to him. Rorty explains that a certain level of solidarity has proven to be a solid basis for a society that is stable and able to secure individuals' safety and prosperity. In fact, the public agreement about this fact is translated into a democratic political system which forces by majority vote every citizen to comply with the system. The result is a constant and dynamic tension between what Rorty calls the private and the public domain.

Medicines, Clinical Research and Clinical Pharmacy Practice

The main purpose of clinical pharmacy research is to investigate whether a specific treatment with medicines has an effect in terms of benefit versus risk (12), i.e. what is the relation between toxicity, which leads to a worsening of a patient's health, and the beneficial effect(s), which lead to an amelioration of the patient's condition? In other words, it is in fact an assessment of the effects of the drug on the patient's autonomy in my ethical terminology. Various pharmacotherapy regimes are evaluated and compared with other therapies and solutions. This approach becomes really complicated when we study interventions for potentially threatening diseases. The so-called "number needed to treat, NNT", which means the number of persons that must be treated to prevent one defined incident in a certain period or to have one successful treatment, should be ideally 1. For many (preventive) therapies the NNT is much higher, up to a few hundred to be treated for many years. Apart from the financial aspects, it means that one person will benefit from this strategy but simultaneously many persons will gain nothing while others definitely experience adverse effects. These effects are never fully quantified (or published?) and balanced against the one "fatal" accident. Is this a matter of ethics, where "to avoid death" is the leading principle?

Such balancing is a culturally dependent process. The standards for such an evaluation are developed by professionals who hopefully present the results as clear choices to the public. At this level there should be a thorough, creative and imaginative discussion. Its outcomes should be accepted on a democratic–political level. So far it seems to be a clear pathway. But then we implicitly assume that every individual will have personal values which fit within the result. The question is, do we accept the result of a group decision if it touches upon our personal life?

A specific clinical study may seem sound and logical, but these ethical issues are always concealed in this process. The ethical issues become larger when practitioners must apply this knowledge in daily life. In other words, how tightly connected are research, knowledge and applicability in pharmacotherapy? How does a general conclusion from a study match with an individual's belief and moral feelings. What type of relation exists between these three interacting elements? It is clear that today we think the responsibility of the practitioners, researchers and politicians is that they should find the greatest possible fit between "general interests" and the individual's sense of justice. That they should even develop provisions for exceptions to the general rules. But can the tension between individualism and solidarity be avoided? Is health gain the most important variable in life compared to other aspects of well-being? For instance employment, or a chance to have children?

THE HEALTH CARE COSTS DILEMMA: ETHICS AND UNEQUAL ACCESS TO HEALTH CARE

To take health care: society decides to limit the health budget, being aware of numerous claims of groups and individuals on public finances. As a consequence, the so-called "right" of the individual for medical treatment is in practice reduced to only that volume that society is prepared to pay for. Take also into account that health, maintaining health and health gain is not exclusively a result of medical treatment. Then it leads automatically to a discussion about the effectiveness of a particular treatment, and to a cost-related protocol for treatment of an individual. To a discussion about priorities: this protocol could even be extended to the field of private behaviour of individuals. Should limited resources be mobilized for people who for their own convenience have a "risky" lifestyle: smoking, wrong food, drinking, not wearing seatbelts? At the same time one could formulate the question: What is the relationship between the well-being of the individual, even with the risky lifestyle, and that of society as a whole? And do not overestimate the impact of (pharmaco)therapy. As we saw before, for many medicines the effect is predictable only on the basis of statistics which do not give any guarantees for effects in individuals. The same reasoning can be applied to "risky" lifestyles.

Democracy and the Role of Protocols and Formularies

Today, protocols are a popular tool to secure "quality". "Quality of outcome" could be translated as: an optimized, predictable and more uniform outcome of a specified intervention. Protocols are designed within a group of professionals and subsequently communicated to the professional domain and to society. "Society" means in our culture the "people", the politicians, the decision-makers. The responsibility of the professionals is to present their choices in a clear and unambiguous way. The responsibility of the politicians is to oversee the total field of requests for public interference in individual lives and to communicate their view to the electorate. The responsibility of the individual is to recognize his often ambiguous role in society. Today a healthy, prosperous individual might simultaneously be a shareholder of a pharmaceutical company, a subscriber to a health-insurance company, a member of a pension fund which invests in the tobacco industry and possibly a patient at the same time. Recognition of these different qualities and responsibilities is very important and will appear to be fundamental for an acceptance of the daily consequences of any decision concerning (personal) health care.

Democracy and Minorities

And what about minorities? Will 51% of the people decide about the access
to health provisions of the other 49%? Is the parliamentary democracy the
modern variation of dictatorship of the majority over the minority? Are
elections a modern non-bloody form of revolution? In a modern society
democracy has many faces. As I pointed out before, it is not only the
parliamentary forum where the decisions, for instance about health care,
are taken. In many countries democracy works on a federal level, on a state
level, in the local community, by means of membership of trade unions, on
the work floor, possibly in the church, in consumer organizations and
through a critical approach to the role of insurance companies and other
health-related industries (13). And the individual plays in this respect
mostly more than one role, and perhaps may even take various standpoints
and at different times show various faces, depending on the forum and
regarding his personal interests. This leads to a result which is much more
complex than the output of a one-dimensional "democratic" decision. The
result will mould into concrete forms of solidarity. An acceptable form of
the limitation of personal autonomy emerges. The result can be seen as the
product of a much more complicated but at the same time more mature
society and should therefore be respected carefully.

In practice, many of us will sometimes face the question of a very expensive medicine or treatment that exceeds by far the health budget. If there has
been discussion and consensus in a practice, in a hospital or in a country
how to act in such a case, then it is not immoral or unethical behaviour to
follow such a protocol, even in the case that one has to abandon treatment
for an individual. It is the result of the balance between the well-being of the
individual and the well-being of society. It still has strongly autonomous
elements in its outcome. It is not the result of a heteronomous process.

The responsibility of pharmacists and doctors is to develop protocols
which respect the patients as individuals and discuss them with all (mentioned) parties involved. Only balanced and updated protocols will protect
health practitioners from unbalanced moral dilemmas. Parallel to this process, clear protocols will show society where the ethical questions are
(14,15). They will force society to take a position, not to hide from its
responsibility and leave it to practitioners. A dynamic process of discussion,
development and updating of the protocols will be necessary to adjust to
changes in time and changes in generations, in other words changes in
culture.

A practical case which demonstrates how difficult it is to apply these
conclusions to the work place was published in a Dutch medical journal at
the beginning of 1998 (16). The use of taxoids for a number of defined
indications appeared to differ from one hospital to another, mainly due to

CASE 2: Pharmaceutical Care

The term "pharmaceutical care" is very confusing for people within and outside the field of pharmacy. The "pharmaceutical care" concept was originally introduced as a clinical protocol to change the role of the (clinical) pharmacist and his place in pharmacotherapy. It tries to organize pharmacotherapy as a more consistent and coherent process (17). The word "pharmaceutical" refers to pharmaceuticals and for that reason many people think that it is something unique to the pharmacy discipline. But in fact it is a multidisciplinary approach to a more consistent form of pharmacotherapy which emphasizes the individual patient, flexibility and evaluation of outcomes from treatments with medicines.

The principle "to restore the individual's autonomy" does not simply translate to "cure" or "make the patient better". It is widely known that patients with a health problem are in the first instance focused on the identification of the nature of that particular problem. The state of "not knowing", the feelings of insecurity, are often very threatening for a person's well-being. The background of this phenomenon is probably based on the belief of Western technology-oriented people that identification of a problem will be the first step in a possible healing process. This attitude requires a certain experience from the health care professional in assessing the patient's feelings, desires and other fundamental elements of that patient's autonomy (18). It implies that the health care professional is properly trained and experienced in communication with the individual's mind and body. When we refer to "informed consent" we must realize that this is the outcome of a complex series of interactions. Psychology as a science and skill supports this complicated and not very well understood process. The relationship between "informed consent" and the autonomy principle is essential. Only a situation of informed consent, of an open and effective communication with a health care practitioner, will create space for decisions that respect autonomy.

Conversely, patients should also be educated to feel responsible and to learn to be a partner in health care, because the respect for other persons applies equally to the health care professional. It will be clear that the health care professional also has rights in respect of his personal autonomy. In the case of a person's request for abortion or euthanasia this fact is clearly recognized by legislation and by professional organizations. To summarize, the patient assessment is not a one-way process. It rather requires the patient's contribution as an autonomous participant.

financial reasons. It was concluded that financial motives were responsible for the *unequal access* of patients to this type of care. It is that inequality which represents the ethical problem.

The Pharmacist

Until this point, individual health problems and the interaction between patient and the medical–diagnostic discipline does not reveal a clear task for the pharmacist. Or it should be mainly as a specialist in toxicology like in the case of an adverse effect of medication being the cause of the problems. Then pharmacy can be considered as a supporting discipline of the physician like radiology, clinical chemistry or microbiology. Under special circumstances and in a proper structure, one could think of a more active role of pharmacists, to alert the physician on possible toxic effects of an existing pharmacotherapy (19). But lack of personal patient data and confidentiality hinder an effective procedure.

If one takes a closer look at responsibilities, the role of the pharmacist starts at the point where, on the basis of clinical assessment of the patient's condition in the broadest sense, a therapy with medicines is considered. Based on my experience, the first priority of the health professional is to stabilize the patient's condition, actually to stop a possible worsening process. The responsibility of the pharmacist overlaps with this principle. It means that he is bound from an ethical point of view to verify whether any pharmacotherapy meets this principle.

In pharmacy practice we know that many medicines harm people instead of curing them (20–22). This is because of medicines being tested and approved on the basis of statistical procedures and outcomes. A medicine is considered as efficacious for example when six out of 10 defined persons show a positive treatment outcome. Does this fact imply that a defined portion of harm is accepted by society as a consequence of "pharmaceutical technology"? Is it the same psychology according to which society accepts thousands of dead and wounded as a consequence of motorized traffic? No, the difference is or might be that in this case pharmacists are educated to minimize these risks of pharmacotherapy. Probably they cannot totally prevent adverse effects, but at least many cases of deterioration of a patient's condition could be avoided if pharmacists would focus on this aspect. This principle sounds rather defensive, but vis-à-vis the potential danger of pharmacologically active substances, "to protect from harm" has through the centuries been a vital task for pharmacists. This is reflected in most national legislation. They all show consistently that the responsibility of pharmacists towards society is still based on toxicity principles. In modern pharmacy practice this essential task is renounced by many practitioners.

What is the Implication of the Word "Care" in Pharmaceutical Care?

In care ethics the patient's needs or wants are the leading principle. Tronto (23) defines care as a continuous process in which four elements can be distinguished: caring about (which can be considered as involvement), to take care of (which implies to take responsibility), care-giving (to take action), and the care-receiving phase (which includes an assessment of the effectiveness). In all of these four steps, there is a role for the pharmacist. Sometimes this will be a minor role, sometimes a more important one. To participate in this process means to have a relationship with patients. They should "take care of" those patients who need extra support with their pharmacotherapy. This relationship should be based on a communicative process as described before (relation to the mind–body), with the mentioned qualifications such as knowledge, training and skills. All based on the assumption that a specific pharmacotherapy is meant to restore the patient's capacity to be him or herself, to restore the maximum achievable autonomy, not to worsen it.

The question is, how can we connect "needs" to the autonomy idea? How do "needs" fit into the informed consent principle? How can we fit professional responsibilities into this process without "taking over" from the patient? First, we must realize that care (giving and receiving) is a continuous process. Care is not a series of isolated happenings. Every moment, every action has a clear connection with the past and coming events. Caring means a period in a person's and patient's life. During this period there will be shifts in dependence: from more dependent to less dependent and back, from more autonomy to less autonomy. During the treatment period there will be a dynamic equilibrium between responsibilities of the care-giver and the care-receiver. The average position or the summation of positions over this time will reflect how the patient's autonomy was respected.

What is the target group for "care" by pharmacists? Health care professionals work in a dynamic environment. A healthy person today can be a patient tomorrow. That implicates that identification of target groups for our "pharmaceutical care" should be performed on a continuous basis. Each group will have specific needs in the field of pharmacotherapy. Assessment of these needs implies that we develop scientific and social criteria and tools to fulfil those needs, together with other health care practitioners. This very dynamic task requires great efforts from pharmacy practitioners (24). If performed well, it will fully occupy the pharmacist and leave hardly any space for commercial or administrative activities.

Pharmacotherapy has become increasingly complicated. When used properly, modern medicines can be very effective. Strong effects also implicate risks. The reduction of risks associated with medicines therefore requires active vigilance and interventions. One can conclude that from an

CASE 3: Euthanasia as an Ethical Question in Pharmacy Practice

A discussion about ethics in pharmacy shifts easily to the field of euthanasia or assisted suicide. A situation where the pharmacist, by the doctor's request, is directly confronted with "applied ethics". Perhaps many pharmacists will feel themselves a little uncomfortable in this matter, because of its material aspect. Pharmacists come from a background where they are not used to making decisions directly connected with death. This is a consequence of pharmacy being one of the "natural sciences". The pharmacy curriculum will therefore have a definitive influence on our future professional attitude. Physicians, being educated at the medical faculty, are more trained and experienced to face situations connected with life and death.

How do we interpret the "principles" to respect autonomy, respect democracy, and avoid harm in this controversial subject? And is this really a new question? Does anyone remember the discussion about sexual morality and oral contraceptives in the 1960s? Or look at the debate about xenotransplantation today, about IVF, the cloning of animals, and experiments with embryos. Many people have the illusion that moral philosophy could be of some use in finding guidelines for practical behaviour. But if we accept that no one philosopher can define a particular truth other than from the cultural perspective, then it is a mistake to look to the moral philosopher for guidance.

However, abandoning the idea of objective truth in ethics does not mean abandoning the standards of consistency and relevance that we uphold in other aspects of our lives. It means for the pharmacist to participate in the public discussion about euthanasia and to bring in personal and professional arguments. But confronted with a request for help, the pharmacist should follow the principles of individual autonomy, respect for (the dignity of) life, not to harm and to respect democratic rules. One could try to simplify the problem by appealing to the law. But the difference between moral reasoning and the way the law interprets active behaviour is that in this case, even passive behaviour can be interpreted as an action. Not doing anything can be an active act. The basic question in euthanasia is how to balance the above-mentioned ethical guidelines. And how to respect the autonomy of the subject, that is to say "the patient" simultaneously with the care-provider. Again a public–professional discussion on how to counter this question should lead to an answer. An answer that is by definition a cultural, place and time dependent guideline for practice.

ethical point of view, an increased attention to chronic patients and those with a high consumption of medicines is a logical pathway to our professional future (25). The pharmacotherapy train could here go off the rails most easily, unless it is manned with skilled and dedicated drivers. Again, this seems a defensive approach. But it is a fact that a passive attitude

---

CASE 4: Clinical Research Projects with Children

Pharmacists are often involved in clinical research. Clinical trials are performed according to the rules of Good Clinical Practice. The trial design has to pass an ethical committee, which will approve the protocol following certain guidelines. This procedure protects the participating individuals (often patients) from harm or unnecessary inconvenience. It is a typical area where the above-mentioned principles can be discussed and balanced against scientific profit.

A more complicated situation arises when people cannot give their consent, like in the case of children. For these cases, the European Agency for Evaluation of Medicinal Products has recently designed specific guidelines. In fact, this area was underdeveloped for many years. Most drugs on the market were routinely applied in the case of children, but were never validated for this use, although one can expect that most drugs will act differently in a child's body from an adult's. In practice, every prescription for a child was a doctor's guess, with a real chance for harm or damage. One of the major problems in clinical practice will be to develop new criteria to test effectivity and efficacy in children. New techniques must be developed and validated, because the reactions of children will differ from those in adults. Long-term studies must show how safety can be guaranteed. Possible influences on growth, cognitive development, sexual development and the influence on the immunosystem should be studied to exclude possible harm in the long term.

For industry, this type of research will have a low priority, due to market arguments. Children are, from a commercial point of view, a minor market. This means for practitioners that they have to be very careful in the prescription and use of medicines which are not adequately tested. The pharmacist can be of assistance in these questions. And if they feel there is a definite need for a specific therapy, or that a particular medicine cannot be missed, then the research question should be brought to a political level. Society should negotiate with professional partners to define its priorities and to find solutions.

towards ongoing therapies potentially creates harmful situations and should therefore be countered.

I estimate that a discussion about the role of the pharmacist as a goal-keeper to avoid negative outcomes of pharmacotherapy would result in great public endorsement today. So let that be the pharmacist's first mission. This conclusion can be translated into practice by promoting a more active role of pharmacists in activities like medication surveillance, proper "communication" about the use of drugs, and the systematic monitoring of adverse effects.

CASE 5: The Future. The Human Genome Project (HGP) and the Practice of Medicine

Until now, "diagnose and treat" has been the leading approach in medicine and pharmacy. This will not change in the case of injuries or infections. But for many other diseases it is expected that medicine will develop finer and much more precise techniques. Today's general approach, based on statistically relevant "evidence-based" medicine, will transform into a "predict and prevent" performance. Not based on group analysis any more, but on molecularly determined biological parameters.

We should realize that many diseases are rare. Also, that the World Health Organization (WHO) has identified some 5000 diseases, of which at least three-quarters have a genetic origin. If one can expect that defects in genetic material, possibly the basis for disease or a limited lifetime, can be identified and repaired, then to cure a specific disease can be more rewarding as an investment in future generations. It even makes it possible to repair the damage and evolutionary "mess" caused by the development of medicine in the past century.

The paradigm will be the change from a "statistics-based" type of medicine to a more individual approach. But is it a real paradigm change? Or is it the application of knowledge that is already available today, but that will be applied on a much larger scale? Are such moments recognizable in history? What about the introduction of insulin? Or the very limited use of penicillin in the 1940s? Probably, the larger scale will confront many practitioners and politicians with ethical questions which have been less relevant in research centres so far. Apart from the cost containment question, the potential use of genetic information can threaten the individual's autonomy and privacy. As we identified, these are strong leading principles in our society and an important base for today's moral standards. It is to be expected that in profit-driven organizations, like insurance companies, the pharmaceutical industry and even in hospitals, company policy will be contrary to these principles. But as we discussed before, an organization consists of individuals who are simultaneously actors in and subject to policies and decisions. They should realize that a responsible organization seeks a public discussion in order to find new standards, acceptable both to industry and to society, health practitioners included. Several countries have already adopted measures to limit the extent to which insurance agents/companies may use genetic information. In the Netherlands, for example, a balance has been reached which safeguards the interests of both insurers and those seeking insurance. Genetic information is disclosed only when unusually large life policies are involved. In the UK the insurance companies have prepared a code of practice which will remove the requirement to report certain types of genetic information in insurance applications.

CASE 6: A Code of Ethics for Pharmacists (26)

A statement about a professional code of ethics for pharmacists was adopted by the council of the FIP in Vancouver in 1997. It summarizes "principles" to comply with in pharmacy practice. The "leading principles" in this statement are unclear. In some cases it refers to "principles" as defined in this chapter. But other statements are very practical, without defining the underlying notion. Such a detailed code for worldwide behaviour will certainly lead to confusion and misunderstanding. In my introduction I have already explained that cultural differences account for the fact that "principles" will manifest themselves in a different way in different places and at different times. For that reason we had better try to define more general principles and leave them to local interpretation.

As we saw, in today's (Western) society the principles of personal autonomy, democracy and solidarity can be seen as essential values. A code of ethics for pharmacists could therefore be based on such a set of ethical principles. The code of ethics should also link to other (health) professionals. My proposal is based on the reasoning that was developed in Cases 1 and 2. A code of ethics for pharmacists could then be formulated as follows:

Continues

Continued

- To recognize and respect the individual's autonomy.
- To follow and respect democratic principles.
- To prevent negative consequences of pharmacotherapy.
- To ensure the best possible treatment.

These principles ask for a cultural and professional translation. Local circumstances will show how the practice of pharmacy can be optimized within this framework. At the same time, the dynamics of this concept are attractive. It will enable pharmacists to discuss professional questions with colleagues, with other health professionals and with society in general.

CONCLUSION

"Abandoning the idea of objective truth in ethics should not mean abandoning the standards of consistency and relevance we uphold in other aspects of our lives" (2). This means that a particular society could agree on "general" principles and rank them in a specific order. A society with a great variety of cultures within its boundaries will find it more difficult to cope with this idea, because the various cultural groups can have different opinions about "essential values" (27). But the individual's autonomy, democracy and solidarity seem to be accepted in a widespread area today. A sharp definition of this basis should be fundamental for a definition of ethics in professional as well as personal life.

ACKNOWLEDGEMENTS

I would like to thank: Jan Flameling (Philosopher), Filosofisch Buro Ataraxia, Amsterdam; Maartje Schermer (Philosopher), Academic Medical Centre AMC, Amsterdam; Steve Hudson (Professor of Pharmaceutical Care, Strathclyde University, Glasgow, UK) for their inspiring discussions and remarks.

REFERENCES

1. Beauchamp TL, Childress YF. Principles of Biomedical Ethics. 4th ed Oxford University Press, 1994.

2. Singer P (ed). *Applied Ethics*. Oxford Readings in Philosophy, 1986.
3. *Ethica Nichomachea. Aristoteles*. Uitg. Kallias b.v.: Amsterdam, 1997.
4. Kant I. *Foundation for the Metaphysics of Morals. Classics of Philosophy*, Pojman LP (ed). Oxford University Press, 1998.
5. *Universal Declaration of Human Rights*, 1948.
6. Leijen A. *Profielen van Ethiek. Van Aristoteles tot Levinas*. Uitg. Coutinho, 1992.
7. Levinas E. *Het Menselijk Gelaat*. Uitg. AMBO: Baarn, 1969.
8. Keij J. *Eenvoudig gezegd: Levinas*. Uitg. Kok Agora: Kampen, 1993.
9. Spreeuwenberg C. Hoe ver reiken de verantwoordelijkheden van de huisarts? *Medisch Contact* 1997; **40**: 281–4.
10. Dupuis HM. Ethische aspecten van de kostendiscussie. *Pharm Weekblad* 1997; **132**: 782.
11. Rorty R. *Contingency, Irony and Solidarity*. Cambridge University Press, 1989, chapter 4; 84.
12. Nilstun T. Clinical pharmacy research: A model for ethical analysis. CMA/ESCP Symposium on Ethical and Economical Aspects of Pharmacotherapy, June 1998, Prague. Department of Medical Ethics, Lund University, Sweden.
13. De Vries G. Fatsoenlijke risicomaatschappij vergt een nieuwe constitutie. *De Volkskrant* 1998; **14 Feb.**
14. Key dilemmas in prescribing and the position of health. *Drug Therapeut Bull* 1997; **35**: 47–8.
15. Nieuwe geneesmiddelen op proef. *Geneesmidd Bull* 1997; **31**: 62–3.
16. Eland IA et al. Verstrekking van taxoiden in 1996: ongelijkheid in de zorg. *Ned Tijdsch Geneeskunde* 1998; **142**: 518. Paclitaxel and docetaxel. *Drug Therapeut Bull* 1997; **35**: 43–6.
17. Hepler CD, Strand LM. Opportunities and responsibilities in pharmaceutical care. *Am J Hosp Pharm* 1990; **47**: 533–43.
18. Schermer M. Autonomie in de gezondheidsethiek en zorgethiek. *Tijdsch Empir Filos* 1997; **21**: 353.
19. Bemt Pvd. *Pharm Weekblad* 1998; **133**: 1269.
20. Lazaron J, Pomeranz BH, Corey PN. Incidence of adverse drug reactions in hospitalized patients. A meta analysis of prospective studies. *JAMA* 1998; **279**: 1200–5.
21. Bates DW. Drugs and adverse drug reactions. How worried should we be? *JAMA* 1998; **279**: 1216–7.
22. Boxtel CJv, Hekster YA, Grootheest ACv. Kennis en bewustwording van ongewenste effecten is noodzakelijk. *Pharm Weekblad* 1998; **133**: 1813.
23. Tronto JC. *Moral Boundaries: A Political Argument for an Ethic of Care*. Routledge: New York/London, 1993.
24. Hudson S. Pharmacy practice research; the student's missing link. *Pharm Weekblad* 1998; **37**: 1384.
25. Rahimtoola H, Timmers A, Dessing R, Hudson S. Target groups for pharmaceutical care. *Pharm World Sci* 1996; 105–13.
26. *Int Pharm J* 1997; **11** (5, Suppl).
27. Heifetz MD. *Ethics in Medicine*. Prometheus Books: New York, 1996.

4

The Ethics of the Drug Discovery and Development Process

ROGER G. BOLTON*

AstraZeneca R&D, Macclesfield, Cheshire, UK

INTRODUCTION

The contribution of new medicines to the improvement of global health and alleviation of disease-related suffering is apparent to all except the most cynical commentators. Since the early evolution of anti-infectives from the dyestuffs industries, and the stimulus given to discovery of such medicines by the needs of the Second World War, the subsequent eras of drug discovery have rolled forward with varying successes and difficulties for different actors in this drama.

In drug discovery there have been several eras, each presenting new ethical challenges, and none more challenging than the "new biology" of the last 15 years, which is still evolving apace.

It is clear that since thalidomide in 1961, a sea-change in approaches to drug development as distinct from discovery has also taken place. No longer were medicines to be developed with minimal pre-clinical testing, and the major concerns being to ensure that quality be maintained consistent with the material first used in humans. Instead the concern has been to apply the optimum pre-clinical and quality testing prior to introduction into

* The views expressed in this chapter are the personal views of the author, and are not necessarily those of his employers or others he may represent.

Pharmaceutical Ethics. Edited by S. Salek and A. Edgar.

humans and to follow this with rigorous testing in the clinic and constant surveillance once marketed. Standards of testing have inexorably risen, and new paradigms have emerged. Yet throughout this process of the evolution of the pharmaceutical industry, an extensive range of ethical issues have had to be addressed, and indeed remain under continuous review. These can be presented in outline as in Table 4.1, and will be discussed and elaborated in the following pages.

In essence they are:

- What should we research on?
- Where is development work best conducted?
- How quickly to progress in a particular development?
- How much to spend on development of new medicines?

Since ethical judgements are made upon the basis of society's normal expectation of what is right and proper, and since modern drug development must by its very nature be a global activity, it is necessary to adopt some form of global ethical framework for a company's operation. On a global basis, however, there is never a way in which this will satisfy the expectations of all the separate subgroups of this global society. One such example is the pressure applied by the gay rights organizations in the 1990s to expedite marketing of new treatments for AIDS without the full requirement for independent and systematic proof of efficacy, which would probably be inconsistent with the expectations of other patient groups such as

Table 4.1 Ethical issues to be faced in drug development

What?

- Selection of research targets
- Selection of candidate drugs

Where?

- Investment
- Returns on investment in R&D
- Non-tariff barriers to introduction of new medicines
- Quality of data
- Preventing exploitation of "soft" regulatory regimes

When?

- Timing of development in relation to laboratory testing (ICH M3)
- Speed of development/cutting corners

How?

- Phasing development to optimize chances of success
- Balancing safety with progress
- Expedited and conditional approval strategies

asthma or heart disease. In this instance the judgements will be specific to the different therapy areas.

In this chapter the "pros" and "cons" of various ethical issues will be discussed and the reader is invited to consider where they would stand faced with the decisions of the various parties involved. The references given are not exhaustive, but reflect the issues in circulation at the time of finalizing this chapter. The very nature of an innovative business requires furthermore that new issues will emerge as scientific breakthroughs are made. Arguably the present time is perhaps the most demanding ever for drug researchers and developers with regard to addressing unprecedented ethical questions. Many of the specific issues concerning the ethics of drug discovery and development are covered in greater detail elsewhere in this book, hence this chapter deals more with the overall subject.

WHAT SHOULD THE INDUSTRY BE WORKING ON?

Research Targets

It is an established observation that those economic systems which do not offer effective intellectual property and a potential for adequate return on investment are not successful in pharmaceutical innovation. However, the very subjects of intellectual property and selection of research targets are often considered controversial in the context of human medicines research. So-called "anti-capitalist" movements have gained some support since the mid-1990s to create forceful opposition to existing economic models, although how the mega-funding of major new medicines developments is to be achieved otherwise is hard to see.

It is often judged that medicine is a special area to which society should not apply normal economic rules. The pharmaceutical industry is expected to work on targets that will never return an investment, and should not exercise its intellectual property in the same manner as in other manufacturing industries so as to support further employment and growth. It is fully accepted that neither research into rare diseases nor those which occur only in socially and economically deprived societies should be excluded, but the ethical dilemma which society must address is how to fund this innovative activity. The economic drivers can be modified. Society in the form of the public sector might fund the activity. Special situations can be created in which compassionate supply, abbreviated testing programmes, or "exceptional circumstances" are designated for so-called "orphan drugs".

What is clear is that no drug development organization should discriminate on the grounds of ethnicity or politics *per se* against a population which is threatened with a public health risk.

A recent report from the Office of Health Economics has similarly advocated a "push-pull" approach to motivate development of medicines and vaccines for neglected diseases that affect less developed countries (1). Recent arrangements by two of the biggest global companies to supply their anti-malarials cheaply or free of charge in Africa via the programmes of the World Health Organization (WHO) (2), and others who have committed to donating to WHO to support treatments in trypanosomiasis (3), are further examples of the response of the innovators to meet special local needs with consideration.

Most companies involved in drug discovery maintain a research and development portfolio that takes account of overall feasibility, economic return and diversity.

Mention may be expected here of the recent action against the South African government's new Medicines Act, but this has nothing to do with selection of research targets. The issue relates to distribution and recognition of globally agreed intellectual property rights rather than development decisions. The press focused on treatments for HIV/AIDS. Here is a scourge of both the developed and the emerging economies. The drug development response has been of amazing benefit to mankind since the pessimistic predictions of the mid-1980s, when the public despaired of a treatment for the virus. The South African interaction has resulted in offers to supply badly needed medicines for HIV/AIDS at prices that the local economy can stand (4), but which would be globally uneconomic. It is however vital that all these medicines reach the patients who need them, and are not traded onwards commercially for financial gain. Hence the global intellectual property agreements have a pivotal role in enabling this type of compassionate supply.

Selection of Candidate Drugs

Having decided upon areas in which to conduct research, drug companies are then faced with issues of how to prioritize the research leads and candidate drugs these discovery programmes create. It is a dilemma with an ethical dimension if a company has a surfeit of opportunities, as much as if it has none. On what basis should a company decide to develop one molecule at the expense of another?

Horrobin (5) has articulated the fact that in order to sustain average industry growth, a company has to introduce each year one new product which will sell around £UK300mn per year for every 1–1.5% it has of the world pharmaceutical market.

Potential return on investment is a product of the overall market size and the impact of a new breakthrough that will determine ultimate market share. A commercial organization has a legal responsibility to its shareholders to maximize the return on its business, hence return on investment has to be the driver. However, this is not inconsistent with an ethical position that offers for licence candidate drugs that it does not intend to commercialize itself. In this respect the discovery is open to development by someone else who considers they can operate profitably. It is also a fact that no company will sustain the costs of patent protection for an invention they consider of no value. Hence they will dispose of the rights either for a small profit or by abandoning the patents if they cannot be sold. Others are always then able to operate in the area, profiting from the original invention.

One real dilemma was creatively addressed by Merck, Sharpe & Dohme (MSD) who discovered the value, in onchocerciasis (African river blindness), of ivermectin, an anthelmintic they wished to commercialize in the developed world for use in veterinary medicine. It would have been economically non-viable to market the product in those countries where it would be useful, yet they carried out the necessary development. Since 1987 ivermectin has been included in the Onchocerciasis Control Programme as the pivotal part of the therapeutic regimen. Ivermectin is being donated worldwide without charge by MSD for treating all persons with onchocerciasis for as long as the drug is needed (6).

A further dilemma can arise when the output of a research programme generates a molecule with activity in a closely related application, or when society shifts the balance of its position between start and fulfilment of a discovery programme. Some applications in reproductive medicine enter this category when an endocrine modulator demonstrates, say, abortifacient properties which would have practical applications, subject to ethical provisos. It may be that the company then has to re-think its position in that target area.

WHERE SHOULD THE INDUSTRY BE PERFORMING R&D?

Laboratory Studies

Recent estimates of the cost of development of a new medicine for treatment of a wide population are around €560mn, costed from the point of selection. The EU research-based Pharmaceutical Industry in 1999 spent an estimated €15bn on R&D (7), of which it is estimated that 25–35% goes into discovery programmes. An estimated 82,500 people were employed in research and development in the EU (8). This discovery activity includes exploratory research into disease mechanisms as well as programmes to discover and evaluate potential lead compounds, several of which will be unsuccessful or lead to candidate drugs which later fail when safety and efficacy testing for marketing approval is carried out. This huge investment in research is clearly a potential benefit to the economies of countries where it is done, but what determines the location of research laboratories or the sites of clinical trials?

Quality of the local research infrastructure and its relevance to the area of research in question is clearly vital. In the developed world science parks have sprung up around centres of academic excellence where the supply of scientists is rich. But equally costs may be higher where there is much competition for limited resources. Since most work other than clinical trials can be conducted in appropriate laboratories irrespective of location, it is normal for each company to grow their own traditional centres of excellence in established technology, with the possible exception of siting centres using completely new technology close to one of the academic centres where the technology was discovered. Cambridge, UK, will certainly hope that this happens in respect of those technologies highlighted in the Human Genome Project. With development of e-working, and broad bandwidth transfer both of data and communications signals, this theory may prove to be fallacious.

However, some governments do recognize the value of R&D investment to their economy, and consequently since these governments also have a control over the policies for pricing and reimbursement of new medicines within the healthcare system, it has long been accepted that local R&D investment may be a factor in determining the approved price of a new medicine. Until around 1990 it was required that foreign manufacturers should repeat their pre-clinical testing in a Japanese laboratory, even though it entailed using the same laboratory-derived strains of rat that had been employed in the country of origin. Such duplication raised its own ethical unacceptability (see below), but served as a deterrent or delay to the introduction of new medicines of foreign origin for some years.

A justification for the repetition of laboratory studies in a second country is the reliability of the data. This raised ethical and legal dilemmas for some years before the establishment of enforceable codes of good laboratory practice and compliance. Until around 1980 it was customary in a number of EU countries to require "confirmatory testing" to be conducted by locally accredited experts. Global standards of good scientific practice are now established and compliance is verified effectively before the data is accepted.

Location of Clinical Trials

In respect of clinical trials, there is greater justification to require local conduct of studies, whenever there are significant differences in disease strain, in medical practice or healthcare provision, in the genetic make-up of populations or significant differences in diet. In the past Japanese clinicians demanded full local clinical trial programmes to be conducted for registration of new products, and as a result differences in normal dosages have developed between Japan and Western countries, popularly perceived to be generally lower in Japan as a consequence of lower mean body weight. Recent studies under the auspices of the International Conference on Harmonization of Technical Requirements for the Registration of New Human Medicines (ICH) have demonstrated in fact that this is unfounded, and the variability of doses of products within Japan is greater than the disparity in general between Japan and the West. Consequently there is no longer a justification for duplication of pivotal studies in different regions, provided that adequate short-term clinical pharmacology studies are conducted to demonstrate that no significant ethnic or population differences would be expected. Confirmatory Phase IIIB or Phase IV clinical work is conducted in various different regional locations to establish those effectiveness parameters which may emerge as a consequence of the many different systems of use of medicines—such work can only be done once the product can be used under conditions approaching normality—i.e. with a proven dose and adequate understanding of the potential adverse reactions profile. Although viewed by some as commercial, it should be said that these studies are an essential part of a responsible and gradual development.

The relevance and rigour of clinical trials is a vital part of the ethics of a study. If the patient is exposed for no worthwhile end, then the risks of that exposure may be considered unjustified. Amongst factors determining study value is the quality of the data. After several worrying instances observed by FDA in the 1970s, where triallists fabricated all or part of the data, or failed to follow the protocol adequately, codes of Good Clinical Practice (GCP) were established. Harmonized under the ICH process in 1995, the guidelines for GCP address the compliance with the protocol, the adequacy of ethical committee opinion, the integrity of the data and its consistency with the final report and the qualifications of the investigators and adequacy of their facilities to perform the particular study. No clinical trial should be started without a favourable opinion from a research ethics committee capable of addressing issues such as those above. In some territories there are no such committees. Failure to comply with GCP guidelines will result in refusal to accept a study in support of an application for marketing approval. Failure of an investigator to conduct studies properly can lead to disbarment from further clinical research.

A further ethical issue in selecting the location for clinical trials is the stringency of the regulatory regimen within a territory. In some there are no rules governing the performance of clinical trials, in others the bureaucracy is oppressive. This does not mean that the one or the other results in a better environment for the patient. However, it is generally recognized that in

BM110
No animal model
No US
Study
UK Approved

practice higher ethical standards lead to higher quality of clinical research. Where there is a more relaxed external regimen each company must decide its required position concerning ethics, and would be ill-advised to consider operating dual standards. Given this safeguard the location of the work can then be independent of the regulatory environment, although the sponsor must ensure that the ethical supervision of patients at the study site is rigorous.

WHEN?

The Ethics of Timing

Drug development is subject to time pressures that arise from the limited time period available for exploitation of newly patented discoveries. Surveys of best practice in the pharmaceutical industry indicate minimum time-scales of 5 to 7 years from identification of preferred candidate through to submission for regulatory approval for marketing. Frequently the time demands are much longer.

The key stages of drug discovery and development are displayed in Figure 4.1. Each stage leads to a decision point at which there is further confirmation of safety and efficacy of the new molecule. At each such milestone a decision is needed on whether it is appropriate to proceed to

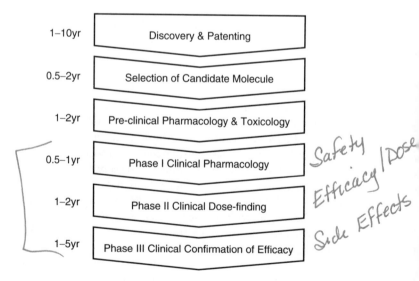

Safety
Efficacy / Dose
Side Effects

Figure 4.1   Drug development steps

further studies. This is not only an investment decision, but also an ethical decision—is the balance of potential benefit to possible risk still acceptable?

Given the potential for failure in scientific studies, observation of unacceptable toxicity, or lack of the required effectiveness, it is clearly financially prudent to minimize risk by conducting all studies sequentially. As a general rule, clinical studies are the most costly investment of a drug development programme, hence if there are any signals of a possible problem these are best received before the later stages of development. In this consideration the investment decision runs in the same direction as the ethical demands of maximum patient safety. However, given the huge costs of development and limited unexpired patent protection at the time of approval for marketing, the need to bring products to market quickly is very real. The ethical considerations of patients' safety must always be set against the attraction of shortcuts in development.

At some point, the initial laboratory studies must lead to a first human exposure. More will be said below concerning the validation of laboratory models, and the ethics of using laboratory animals. However, there is now international consensus between the experts in the three major regions, via the ICH process, as to the acceptable packages of laboratory studies to be satisfactorily completed before human exposure is allowed (9). Human exposure must likewise be progressive from low-risk subjects able to give fully informed consent ultimately to a realistic population of patients who are probably less healthy, and may in some circumstances be less able to give satisfactory consent. Children would normally not be exposed to a new molecule until after confirmation that the new drug had shown benefits in adult patients.

Another important consideration in clinical development is the rate of expansion of patient recruitment, coupled with the resources of a sponsor to monitor adequately the conduct of all centres of trials. In Phase III studies in which the general patient population is exposed to the new product, the rate of recruitment cannot be allowed to outstrip the capacity to gather and evaluate ongoing results for new signals.

Accelerated development could be achieved by a contraction of timescales by a telescoped process; however, this can never be at the cost of an unacceptable risk to patients. Some patient groups, notably those representing AIDS patients, have applied pressure for companies to bring products to market before completion of the normal full testing programme. This is clearly a risky option—the effective burden of ethics, liability and potential damage to the prospects for an otherwise worthy new drug all rest upon the shoulders of the sponsoring company. However, it is recognized that there will be circumstances when an accelerated development is justified, with either a curtailed or a telescoped programme of studies. Clearly under such circumstances the justification of each decision must be well documented.

Exceptional Circumstances

In situations where there is significant unmet medical need, it is justified to consider ways of advancing the access in the marketplace to a potential new treatment. Government regulators have evolved various principles to encourage such acceleration. These are variously labelled, but in general relate to:

- **accelerated review** by the regulators, although still demanding a complete and comprehensive testing programme prior to authorization ("priority review").
- **authorization** on the basis of an incomplete testing programme (e.g. Phase I & II clinical, but no Phase III), subject to favourable scientific assessment of the results, and conditional upon submission of further agreed testing within a defined time-scale ("conditional authorization").
- **in the case of rare diseases**, authorization on the basis of a testing programme less extensive than for other therapeutic areas. The scarcity of patients for study renders participation by equivalent numbers of subjects unrealistic ("orphan drug").

In some circumstances a combination of these exceptional procedures may be applied. In every case there must be seen to be an exceptional medical need for new treatments in life-threatening or seriously debilitating illnesses.

SPECIAL ETHICAL TOPICS IN DRUG DISCOVERY AND DEVELOPMENT

A number of specific topics not covered elsewhere deserve at least a passing mention in this chapter.

The Use of Laboratory Animals

The pharmaceutical industry has long been under attack from those who challenge the ethics of testing new medicines in laboratory animals before human beings. The critics argue variously that the rights of animals are the same as those of humans, or that the results of such experiments are not predictive of effects in humans. Some groups defend these extreme views with threats, even actual physical violence to those whom they view as connected with animal studies.

To deal with these two objections separately, the former depends on a discussion of fundamental beliefs and priorities concerning the sanctity of life and health. Here the ethical judgement has to revolve around the perceptions of society in its largest part, that the human being is special and that a reasonable amount of animal testing is a wise and valuable step prior to exposing a human being to a new risk. Such testing must clearly be conducted with attention to animal welfare and the minimum of pain or distress.

As to the validity of animal models, there is much experience affirming that small mammals will reflect potential effects in the human to a worthwhile degree. Much research is being conducted by toxicologists and pharmacologists to validate models that use isolated enzymes, membranes, tissue or non-mammalian organisms, and there has been significant progress in establishing such new systems. However, at present levels of understanding it remains the considered judgement of a majority of the scientific community that some work in whole animals is an essential step prior to human exposure because such work is capable of making a valid prediction. It is essential to consider how the many isolated body systems might interact in their response to a potential new drug. Biomedical scientists have no desire to persist in unnecessary animal testing, it is extremely costly and even though such procedures are designed always to minimize suffering of the animals, those who work with animals are always concerned for their welfare. Both scientists and non-scientists share the opinion that appropriate testing is a wise precaution.

Clinical Studies in Special Risk Groups

Although, as indicated above, it is beholden upon a company with a medicine under development to defer studies in higher-risk patients until there is firmer evidence of safety and effectiveness demonstrated in normal patients, companies have nonetheless been criticized for preferring to contraindicate high-risk patients rather than generate data with the increased safety risk. Some years ago FDA established a rule to ensure that data was generated on all sections of the target population without discrimination.

With the increased concern of paediatricians that their armamentarium was limited unless they took upon themselves to make off-label use, US Congress took on board in the FDA Modernization Act of 1997 (FDAMA) an earlier text called "The Better Pharmaceuticals for Children Act", and offered incentives for companies carrying out work in response to an FDA request to generate data in children. This addressed the need when a paediatric indication was economically non-viable. Initiatives are now emerging in both the EU and Japan that will press companies to generate more data in children. Special trial design considerations are required, particularly in very young children, such as minimal use of blood sampling and avoidance of any procedure for trial purposes that would upset or distress the child. Similarly a cautious approach to dose progression is essential, since a very fine balance exists in the public mind between de-priving children of access to medicines and exploiting them in medical experimentation.

A similar dilemma exists concerning use of medicines in pregnancy. Some medical conditions spontaneously improve in pregnancy, but many do not and require ongoing treatment. Alternatively a patient may be established on medication and be likely to become pregnant—should they take contra-ceptive precautions or is the safety acceptable? However, the human foetus is known to be sensitive to exogenous compounds, and safety of *both* mother and baby is paramount. Clinical studies in pregnancy, and the collection of data from pregnant women, have to be on a case-by-case basis, subject to a very careful assessment of benefits and risk. As always, adequate informed consent is essential. The potential risk to the individuals is hard to balance against the potential longer-term benefits to society or the wider patient population.

Surrogate Markers

In order to expedite access to new medicines, reduce costs and minimize the use of both human and laboratory animal exposure during development, the use of surrogate markers or "end-points" is frequently considered in both situations. The ethical dilemma here is the balance between greater efficiency in evaluation and the risk that the surrogate may be inadequately predictive of the effect under study.

The debate applied to laboratory animal testing procedures has been elaborated above. Since animal studies are themselves relatively short, a matter of days, weeks or for a "lifetime study" months, the benefits of using surrogates relate to avoiding the use of animals at all. It is the prevailing ethical view today that if in doubt, the whole animal is the better predictor before proceeding to humans. However, in the selection between different potential candidate molecules, there is extensive use of surrogate indicators in order to reduce studies in live animals. This comparison of "like-with-like" is presumed to be acceptable provided there is good validation of the marker opposite the target human system.

In clinical trials the term "surrogate" usually refers to a molecular marker of a disease state, indicating efficacy. However, the established blood bio-chemistry and haematological techniques to indicate potential adverse effects are also effectively surrogate indicators. Surrogates are used particu-larly in the study of chronic diseases in which observable clinical effects may be delayed for months or years, such as HIV infections and some forms of cancer. Levels of PSA (prostate specific antigen) in prostate cancer and CD4 counts or HIV-1 RNA as a marker of the development of AIDS are typical. Changes in these markers are correlated with subsequent improvement in the disease *per se*. The ethical debate revolves around whether it is right to place products on the market claiming efficacy before a statistically relevant demonstration of improved clinical symptoms. For the reasons outlined above under "exceptional circumstances", groups representing AIDS patients lobbied hard in the early 1990s to expedite access to new treatments via approval on the basis of improved CD4 counts as the sole efficacy measure.

Pharmacogenomics

The study of the human genome and its products as they relate to drug discovery and development (pharmacogenomics), the study of DNA sequence variation as it relates to differential drug response (pharmacogenetics) and the study of DNA sequence variation as it relates to the causes of disease (disease genetics) are tools which have developed dramatically in recent years. Consequently these new applications have raised special concerns of an ethical nature.

Probably the most important ethical consideration is the protection of the personal data resulting from studies. The opportunities that could arise for discrimination in respect of insurance risk or long-term fitness to work have been much debated, and extend the scope of application of opinions addressed to HIV status from diagnostic tests. The risks of discrimination or blackmail are clearly minimized by the normal practice of anonymization of samples taken for genetic analysis. When they are de-personalized and any linking code is destroyed, then adverse findings cannot be correlated back to the donor. However this raises another potential ethical concern, namely that certain findings might be of value in preserving or protecting the health of the individual, and if anonymized, the donor of the sample cannot be reached by their physician for appropriate counselling or treatment.

As with many other ethical dilemmas this has to be dealt with by the adequacy of the informed consent, which in this instance does not only set out the value of the research, the number of examinations, blood samples, etc. required, and the physical risks and inconvenience faced by the subject who consents to the trial. The procedures for anonymization and the resultant protection and obstruction to follow-up are also explained so that the subject is clear about what might or might not happen as a result of sampling.

A further potential issue relates to the possibility, in a fast-moving area of science, that the potential for studies runs ahead of an ongoing experiment. Samples taken under informed consent may present opportunities for further studies as a result of new discoveries. On the one hand it appears unethical to waste a sample which is the generous gift of a donor, yet a consent must exist which covers the new experiment. This must be addressed either by an adequate form of "open-ended consent" agreed as being ethical in its scope, or otherwise the donor or their legal representative must be contacted for further consent. In all these studies it is better when the interests of a patient are addressed by their own doctor, with the researcher providing the requisite information and background for the ethics committee and the informed consent. Thereafter, the researcher will be presented with an anonymized sample for analysis within the bounds of the consent. If any feedback of findings from the researcher to the patient is justified, the doctor again should decide and deliver any actions to the patient in their best interests.

Research Using Human Cells

In addition to the genetic studies in humans, there may occasionally be a need for investigations in vitro using functional human tissue or involving tissue samples from biopsy or secondary to elective surgical procedures. Until the last decade a view did prevail in some circles that tissue removed post-mortem or through elective surgery might freely be used for bona fide medical research. Recent events in the United Kingdom have demonstrated that the general perception of society does not share this view, and that any procedure involving human tissue must have the consent of the relevant concerned parties. Although there is little doubt that most relatives would support efforts to combat the disease that has afflicted one of their family, this does not obviate the need for specific consent.

CONCLUSION

This chapter has sought to focus on those aspects of drug discovery and development which will not have been the subject of other chapters in this book. Hence many general ethical issues applicable to clinical trials have not been addressed here. Neither does this chapter address systems for research ethics committees, the Declaration of Helsinki, or the active debate in the institutions of the European Union surrounding fitness to grant informed consent within the recently adopted Directive on Clinical Trials. These will all be dealt with elsewhere. It is also accepted that space does not permit other deeper ethical questions to be addressed, such as how the benefits of drug development are best harnessed and applied.

Continues

Continued

Whilst few disagree with the important contribution of the pharmaceutical industry to worldwide human health, the existence of stern critics challenges the industry to think carefully about each ethical decision it makes. In respect of studies involving human and animal welfare it is essential that the scientist or doctor can defend themselves against challenges of being arrogant or unfeeling. In every instance the potential for benefit must be evaluated against the risks or potential for suffering. Whenever human subjects are involved, the need for properly obtained informed consent and a favourable opinion from a properly constituted independent ethics committee is essential, and proper justification for all studies in animals must be given. Gratuitous exposure of patients or animals is avoided in all responsible companies, and the codes of Good Clinical Practice and Good Laboratory Practice are rigorously applied. These codes in themselves require studies to be properly justified within a specific protocol and the conduct of all work must be demonstrably compliant with the codes. It is an accepted view within the industry that good ethics encourages better quality science.

SUGGESTED FURTHER READING

Where?

de Silva J. Site selection for clinical trials. *Drug Inf J* 1998; **32**: 1257S–8S.

When?

Getz KA, de Bruin A. Breaking the development speed barrier: assessing successful practices of the fastest drug development companies. *Drug Inf J* 2000; **34**: 725–36.
Clemento A. New and integrated approaches to successful accelerated drug development. *Drug Inf J* 1999; **33**: 699–710.

Special Risk Patients

Simar MR. Paediatric development: the ICH focus on clinical investigations in children. *Drug Inf J* 2000; **34**: 809–19.
Milne C-P. The paediatric studies initiative. In *New Drug Development: A Regulatory Overview*, 5th edn, Mathieu M (ed). Tufts Centre for the Study of Drug Development: USA, 2000.
Hoet JJ. The ethics, vigilance and rationale for conducting clinical trials during pregnancy. In *European Conference Publications*, Fracchia GN, Haavisto KH (eds), 1996; 175–81.

Levine RJ. Research involving pregnant women as subjects: ethical considerations. In *European Conference Publications*, Fracchia GN, Haavisto KH (eds), 1996; 181–8.

Surrogates

Chuang-Stein C, deMasi R. Surrogate endpoints in AIDS drug development: current status. *Drug Inf J* 1998; **32**: 439–48.
Fleming TR. Surrogate endpoints in clinical trials. *Drug Inf J* 1996; **30**: 545–51.
Berman RE. FDA approval of antiretroviral agents: an evolving paradigm. *Drug Inf J* 1999; **33**: 337–41.

Pharmacogenomics

Wattanapitayakul S, Schommer JC. The human genome project: benefits and risks to society. *Drug Inf J* 1999; **33**: 729–35.

General

Lyons DJ. Use and abuse of placebo in clinical trials. *Drug Inf J* 1999; **33**: 261–4.
Lin MH. Ethical considerations in clinical trials: an international perspective. *Drug Inf J* 1998; **32**: 1293S–7S.

REFERENCES

1. Kettler H. *Narrowing the Gap between Provision and Need for medicines in Developing Countries*. Office of Health Economics: London, 2001.
2. Scrip, 10th May 2001. Article S00709034 F. PJB Publications Ltd, 2000.
3. Scrip, 8th May 2001. Article S00708508 F. PJB Publications Ltd, 2001.
4. Scrip, 21st May 2001. PJB Publications Ltd, 2001.
5. Horrobin DF. *J R Soc Med* 2000; **93**: 341–5.
6. Goa KL, McTavish D, Clissold SP. *Drugs* 1991; **42**: 640–58.
7. *The Pharmaceutical Industry in Figures: 2000 Edition*. European Federation of Pharmaceutical Industries & Associations: Brussels, p. 21.
8. Ibid, p. 9.
9. ICH M3: "Timing of Pre-clinical Studies in Relation to Clinical Trials". The official website for ICH, http://www.ifpma.org/ich5.html

5

Informed Consent: Reconsideration of its Structure and Role in Medicine

JAN PAYNE

Institute for Human Studies in Medicine, First Medical Faculty,
Charles University, Prague, Czech Republic

ABSTRACT

This chapter deals with informed consent as a new and rather complicated structure of social relations between doctor and patient. Medicine has developed it quite recently, and this brief history, with some putative reasons for the delay, are mentioned first, then informed consent is analyzed and divided into three levels of decision-making. It must be taken into account that informed consent is a dilemma, and that there is thus no proper general decision valid for every case.

Keywords: Autonomy; Decision-making; Dilemma; Informed consent

HISTORICAL REMARKS

The concept known as "informed consent" did not emerge until the second half of the twentieth century and, as historians suggest, the professional

Pharmaceutical Ethics. Edited by S. Salek and A. Edgar.

literature applied it first in 1957 in the USA with regard to issues of law (1). The proper discussion of informed consent began, however, later in the seventies, while it is still increasing in importance. At the present time it is a key category in medicine, without which nothing can be done for the patient. Similarly, this category is also a basic precondition for any research with human beings. All this suggests that medicine has been going through a profound change, which amounts to a shift in its paradigm as Thomas Kuhn uses the term (2).

What is actually going on? We must take into account that before the Second World War physicians relied on their own judgment and paid little attention to the judgment of their patients regarding treatment. In other words, the patient's autonomy was ignored, which is rather amazing since other realms of modern society had gone through transformation in the direction of greater emphasis on the self-determination of each person much earlier, and this shift had found its expression in the notion of human rights. Yet medicine was slow to change until recently: actually even the Code of the World Medical Association adopted in 1947, which is otherwise noble, does not refer to autonomy at all. An emphasis on autonomy hand-in-hand with the demand for disclosure of relevant medical facts to the patient makes up the core of informed consent as it has been elaborated in recent years.

We might be haunted by the question of how it could happen that such an important category as that of autonomy, with the doctrine of human rights accompanying it, could had been omitted so thoroughly in medicine, although in other social realms the opposite prevailed. What is the reason for such neglect, which appears to be in conflict with the traditional humane ambitions of medicine?

At least three factors seem to have played a role in delaying the acceptance of autonomy in medicine so far.

(i) First, we must be aware that medicine as we know it is not the single possible, necessarily developed and therefore "general" medicine valid for all times; actually there were other movements of physicians and healers who competed with the school of *Hippocratics*, and even in Greece this tradition was not the strongest among them. Nonetheless, this stream of medicine has become dominant and now represents the common and customary way of medical treatment. Yet it still bears traits of its origins, one of which is its reliance on the two and a half thousand year old Hippocratic Oath, which is still being sworn in some way. This Oath, as well as other parts of the *Corpus*, lack any hint at self-determination bestowed upon the patient and consequently no imperative protecting her/his free will (3). Although we have taken up this Oath almost literally, the difference between contemporary and ancient medicine is dramatic and deep. The Greek political system was based on slavery, and slaves by definition were deprived of self-determination, so that to treat them humanely meant to skip such a moral tenet. Actually, medicine has preserved that failure and with some exaggeration it might be argued that the slave relationship between the patient and the doctor has not entirely vanished from medicine so far.

(ii) Second, we should take into account that the medieval period, lasting about 10 centuries, also exerted a considerable impact on medicine. Medicine was shaped at that time by religious philosophy and also by the dogmatic assumption of God the Creator, who plotted everything beforehand in forms. The entire being was shaped with regard to the ultimate Good, while goods derived from it served as prototypes for each part of the whole. Health then, of course, could not fall out of this scheme and physicians endowed with education were acquainted with the proper norms, whereas lay patients were naïve. Because of this, they were doomed to obey the instructions and directives of their doctors, and if they disagreed with those orders, were necessarily considered either mad or dull (4). So, if any conflict occurred, the patient was *a priori* wrong and the doctor was relieved of any burden of paying attention to the patient's whims. There was thus no room for negotiation between the patient and the doctor, and hence informed consent simply did not come into it.

(iii) Third, we cannot forget that people in general are scared by liberty if it exceeds accustomed borders. As some philosophers have pointed out (5), true liberty is an abyss inciting dizziness and many, or perhaps the majority, have always avoided it. Only a minority of people acquainted with what autonomy means have felt a commitment to plead for it, despite all the menaces and vexations it entails. This fear of liberty, or rather the sheer anxiety of facing it, is probably another important reason why autonomy was so long ignored by medicine. Doctors dislike cases in which their intentions clash with the intentions of their patients, and tend to dispose of such strife. Yet there is no other way out now. This rather post-modern approach resembles, due to its doubt about any firm Archimedean point, classical relativism and skepticism. Skepticism, however, can still serve as a starting point for a lofty ethics, and this ethics, despite its dire connotations, is probably the sole one suitable for the future pluralistic world (6).

These three factors influenced modern society, so that it postponed discussion on autonomy until recently. Actually, until the time when American lawyers coined the term "informed consent" for cases of clinical practice, where the rights of patients seemed to be encroached upon. A further incentive for debate about this topic came from the profound misuse of human research during the Second World War, regulated later by the Nuremberg Code (1948) as well as other codes such as that of Helsinki (1964), with later improvements. From these different vantage points an ardent debate on patient self-determination was launched.

ANALYTICAL REMARKS

Since it is based on self-determination, informed consent represents a complex and complicated structure of social relations (necessarily since autonomy itself is an enigmatic issue). The structure of informed consent comprises a series of decisions, within which we can distinguish three levels. However, these levels are nonetheless interwoven, and the distinction serves merely didactic purposes.

Competence of the Patient

The initial decision, which is a precondition for others, concerns whether the patient is able to make decisions at all, and if so, how competent they are. When the patient lacks this capacity to make a choice (an extreme form would be coma), autonomy is lost and informed consent is not attainable. Certainly medicine must reckon with such cases, and work out a system of surrogate decision-makers (7), but this strategy is not informed consent as such.

The main problem is how to assess the degree of capacity to make decisions when it is to some extent impaired due to either "cultural" background, like poor education, or "natural" causes, such as various diseases. This evaluation is of the utmost importance, and can be considered an "ethical diagnosis". It is not directly feasible by the ordinary means of getting knowledge, since it deals not with reality but with potentiality. Potentiality was abandoned, however, by the sciences from the very beginning, while thinking about it was refuted as bare raving. Yet moral judgment must take potentialities and possibilities into account, since guilt is to be imputed only to the one who could have acted otherwise. In contrast with that judgment which deals with past events, the task of assessing future events is much more difficult, while this is just what we must do in assessing the competence of a patient to make decisions about her/himself.

It may be useful here to propose a putative structure of that competence which is a mere possibility, and which may be rendered by the name "project" or simply called the will (8). What needs to be reckoned with is that the project can be approached solely by the peculiar method of interpretation, known as hermeneutics. Hermeneutics treats intentions and deliberate motives in their complexity as its proper target of scrutiny, and this discipline is thus best equipped to assess also the competence to make decisions in others (9). In other words, medicine is also hermeneutic by its character, and this discipline, with its knowledge and skills, should be incorporated into the curriculum too.

Another way of assessing competence to make decisions is associated not with a sufficient but with a necessary condition. Certainly decisions are not made beyond reality, and can be located with regard to recent scientific discoveries in the most developed parts of the brain, which are the frontal lobes (10). Different kinds of lesions of this frontal cortex indeed cause impairment of the ability to make decisions, and this clinical observation can also be employed in the assessment of competence as mentioned above. We can but hope that in the future some more sophisticated theory about the function of the frontal lobes in relation to making decisions will be formed (11). In any case, normally working frontal parts of the brain are a necessary condition for proper decision-making.

One remark that must be made is *katexochén* ethical. Ethics deals with unpredictable events, which means we are to think in terms of a future bifurcation where the proper direction of development is not known in advance. To solve this puzzle means to have some presumption, be it unconscious or conscious. Conscious presumptions should be preferred, which requires us to reflect on what we feel. This brings us to the question of whether we ought to presume either incompetence or competence. A human approach gives a direct answer: we should in every case assume the full competence of the patient unless we have proof to the contrary.

Conflict of Principles

The next decision which is accompanied by much confusion concerns the clash of moral norms, known as a dilemma (12). A dilemma appears when we have a code with two principles which are contrary to each other and thus prompt us to opposing actions. In attempting to elucidate this obscurity we need to distinguish two branches of ethics: the ethics of dilemma and the ethics of temptation (13). Temptations come about when there is a conflict between inclinations and principles, whereas the collision of two principles is a dilemma proper, which has a peculiar regimen of coping. It must be stressed that there is no general way of solving dilemmas. This runs counter to our acquired habits of dispatching every problem by some general rule. Sciences are based on just such regularities, and our education deals almost entirely with sciences, so that we have scanty notions about other powers of reason.

Actually there is the power of judgment, which can be rendered also by terms like "common sense", "prudence" and "taste". All these terms are translations of the Greek word *"fronesis"*, deeply reflected on already by Aristotle (14). Kant later postulated that this art of judgment, tied with concrete cases, evades grasp by abstract concepts, as well as any chance of being taught. Those who lack it remain stupid (*dumm*), despite their possibly ample education (15). Reason, however, is based on judgment, which is the capability to attach some general term to a unique event, and this is just what we need for coping with dilemmas in medicine (16).

Modern health care is endowed with codes that comprise conflicting principles, and its dilemmas must be solved in every case anew. In other words: *there are no two cases of dilemmas similar enough so that a decision in one case can be transferred to the other.* Among such principles we must point out two: the principle of non-maleficence (in the weak form) and the principle of beneficence (in the strong form) on the one hand (17) and the principle of autonomy on the other hand. They come into accord only by chance, which means that the opinion of the doctor is rarely identical with the opinion of the patient (18). Informed consent then serves to reconcile this quarrel (19).

Some might argue that having accepted autonomy we ought to let the patient (patient as client and customer) make decisions about everything. Such a tendency is quite common, since doctors are prone to avoid unpleasant risky conflicts of two rules and to prefer only one of them. Yet it is in principle wrong, since decisions are always dependent on information which can never be complete. Medicine embraces such a vast amount of knowledge that it is not amenable to mediation in real clinical practice, where the staff are busy and overloaded. A physician is therefore compelled to make a selection of what should be articulated, which necessarily requires evaluation according to some criteria and measures. All information is exposed to subjective bias (of course, either immoral or moral), and thus absolute objectivity can never be achieved (20).

Being charged to choose how much information to tell to the patient, physicians are faced with two possibilities. Either to make that choice without any evaluation and therefore at random by some kind of lottery, which would be a bizarre option in medicine, or to pursue some criterion of good, which means that the patient is necessarily in some sense manipulated, although it may often be with the best aims. Obedience to the Hippocratic precept *"primum nil nocere"* is thus always present, even though autonomy of the patient has been accepted and informed consent should lead to the decision which of these principles should prevail in concrete cases.

It is worth mentioning here that we must maintain a distinction (actually artificial) between two kinds of information. Information either (a) considering past treatment, in regard to what in fact has been done (diagnosis) and has happened, which can quite easily be precise and which, according to the moral standard, ought to be exhaustive in every sense or (b) in advance and about the possible consequences (prognosis), which is always only conjecture based on some statistical data and which cannot but be influenced by the moral attitude of the doctor her/himself.

Although in clinical practice it is rather difficult to separate both these procedures (medical treatment may be resumed at any time), we must try to since the latter necessarily requires assessment and may in some cases be either postponed or even dropped due to an intention not to harm, whereas the former is out of dispute and simply must be obeyed (regarding the principle of veracity).

Conflict of Interests

The final decision comparable with decisions in other spheres of social life is the one that we make when concluding a contract. Contracts are often preceded by some conflict, yet it is the conflict of interests of two persons and not of principles in the heart of one person, as in the case above. (A conflict of interests or propensities in one person is usually called neurosis, and must be medically treated.)

As to principles, we encounter here only the principle of autonomy and the conflict comes about due to the clash of two autonomous beings. This collision must be overcome by negotiation and through compromise, which indeed requires decisions on both sides. Of course informed consent is also a result of such bargaining, which means that even when decisions have been made about competence (competence is considered perfect) and autonomy (autonomy is regarded as prevailing), the doctor can still waive one-sided assent.

Medical treatment, however, is such that bargaining between the doctor and the patient is never finished unless the patient recovers. Rarely do we write a document that lays down an achieved agreement (for example, before an operation or other radical treatment) and is a legal fixation of a temporary opinion. The remaining negotiation, with its moments of agreement, is in contrast *par excellence* moral and must be permanent (21). Actually we can call this part of the informed consent "shared decision-making", which is a lively story with an open end. The general assumption is that no intervention in medicine is permitted unless this condition is fulfilled.

It is fair to mention that proper negotiation is valid only for clinical practice, while in medical research there is a slightly different model, since the experimental subject cannot discuss possible alternatives in research protocols as is the case in treatment. Some negotiation in research is delegated to the research ethics committee, which is the proper *raison d'être* and mandate of its establishment. In contrast, the experimental subject or patient (in therapeutic studies) is confronted with the mere "block" option of "yes/no" (here we can conceive of consent as an assent uttered by the experimental subject).

Pharmaceutical Ethics

Despite this peculiarity of research we still should reckon with informed consent as a contract between two sovereign persons who enjoy autonomy and who must always negotiate about possible compromises on both sides. In a pluralistic society it is absolutely impossible to command someone to do something. In fact, the etymology of the English word "consent", which has been derived from the Latin word "consensus", refers to agreement as a mutual approval. Proper consent is thus never a one-sided confirmation based on one-sided information, which is better called assent to something. On the other hand, we should never forget the former levels of decision-making, which can compromise any possible agreement between the patient and the doctor. Medical examination may at any moment reveal new details that prompt us to correct our former conclusions.

CONCLUSION

Informed consent has three phases of decision, which follow one after another, yet they are all made usually at once. This structure of social relations is not as new as it may seem. In fact, everybody has had some experience of it, since an almost identical structure can be found in the relationship between either parents and children or teachers and pupils. Despite the fact that this relationship contradicts logic and, as a paradox, runs counter to any way in which it can be carried out, everybody has been brought up in this manner. Perhaps research on these three classical social attachments will be mutually fertilizing, so that some time in the future we shall gain more knowledge about them.

How to summarize the whole problem of informed consent? Medicine is here confronted with a question lacking any simple answer. We may conjecture that the meaning of it is to give us a lesson about how to live with questions lacking answers, how to be open to the future and particularly to others. In this sense, thinking about informed consent has a moralizing impact on our character and should be promoted everywhere in medicine.

REFERENCES AND NOTES

1. Beauchamp TL. Informed consent. In *Medical Ethics*, Veatch RM (ed). Jones and Bartelett: Boston, 1989; 175–7, 198.
2. Payne J. The nature and the future of medicine. In *Medicine Today and our Image of Man*. FEAMC: Prague, 1996; 72–4.

3. Reiser SJ. Ethical dimensions of the physician–patient relationship through history. In *Ethics in Medicine*, Reiser SJ, Dyck AJ, Curran WJ (eds). MIT Press: Cambridge, MA, 1985; 5–9.

4. Faden RR, Beauchamp TL. *A History and Theory of Informed Consent*. Oxford University Press: Oxford, 1986; 56–7, 63–4.

5. Kierkegaard S. *Der Begriff Angst*. Eugen Diederichs Verlag: Dusseldorf, 1958; 161–3.

6. A quite successful attempt to base ethics on skepticism strong enough to defy any other skepticism about itself has been made by the German philosopher Weischedel. Weischedel W. *Skeptische Ethik*. Suhrkamp: Frankfurt am Main, 1976; 179–208.

7. Moreno JD. Who's to choose? Surrogate decision making in New York State. Hastings Centre Report 1993; **23** (1): 5–11. Blutstein J. The family in medical decision making. Hastings Centre Report 1993; **23** (3): 6–13.

8. Ricoeur P. *Freedom and Nature* (transl: Kohak EV). Northwestern University Press: New York, 1966; 41–55.

9. Payne J. *Hermeneuticka etika*. Triton: Prague, 1955; 18–37.

10. It must not be forgotten that the frontal cortex is part of more complex circuits, including particularly the mediodorsal nucleus of the thalamus and corpus striatum. Creuzfeld OD. *Cortex Cerebri: Strukturelle and funktionelle Organisation der Hirnrinden*. Springer-Verlag: Berlin, 1983; 310–22.

11. Damasio AR. *Descartes' Error: Emotion, Reason and the Human Brain*. Avon Books: New York, 1994; 212–22, 253–60.

12. Beauchamp TL, Childress JF. *Principles of Biomedical Ethics*. Oxford University Press: Oxford, 1989; 4–6.

13. Hartmann N. *Ethik*. Walter de Gruyter: Berlin, 1962; 212–4.

14. Aristotle. *The Nicomachean Ethics* (transl: Welldon JEC). Macmillan: New York, 1906; 183–6 (Book V, chapter 6).

15. Kant I. *Kritik de Reinen Vernunft*. Georg Weiss: Heidelberg, 1884; 166 (Von der transcendentalen Urteilskraft ubehaupt: note).

16. The reason is endowed with a unique power which is the art of judgment and which typically evades rules for its application on concrete cases since such rules would again require other rules for their application and this would be an infinite regress. Comp: Caygill H. *Art of Judgment*. Basil Blackwell: Oxford, 1989; 11 (chapter 1).

17. These two principles are equivalents of the Hippocratic precept "*primum nil nocere*". Comp: Faden RR, Beauchamp TL. *A History and Theory of Informed Consent*. Oxford University Press: Oxford, 1986; 61–3.

18. Dworkin G. *The Theory and Practice of Autonomy*. Cambridge University Press: Cambridge, 1989; 25.

19. A typical example of such reconciliation is the DNR order (do not resuscitate), which assumes that both the team of doctors and the patient along with her/his relatives agree about forgoing further treatment. Comp: Reich WT (ed). *Encyclopaedia of Bioethics*. Macmillan/Simon and Schuster: New York, 1995; 569–70.

20. There are attempts to propose informational, professional and IAIC standards which again represent some kind of presumption. Comp: Beauchamp TL. Informed consent. In *Medical Ethics*, Veatch RM (ed). Jones and Bartelett: Boston, 1989; 184–6.

21. Ibid; 183–4.

6

Clinical Trials of Pharmaceuticals: Ethical Aspects

OLIVIER CHASSANY[1,*], MARTIN DURACINSKY[2] AND ISABELLE MAHÉ[3]

[1]Délégation à la Recherche Clinique, Assistance Publique—Hôpitaux de Paris, 75010 Paris, France [2]Department of Internal Medicine, Saint-Louis University Hospital, 75010, Paris, France[3]Department of Internal Medicine, Lariboisière University Hospital, 75010 Paris, France

SUMMARY

Since the Nuremberg Code in 1947, several codes of human rights in medical research have been released. The best known and current reference guideline is the Declaration of Helsinki. Three major principles are emphasized, i.e. respect for patients, beneficence and justice. Respect of the patient to accept or not participate in a trial; the constraints and presumed risks must be acceptable for patients included in a study; and vulnerable subjects should not participate in studies. The investigator is responsible for obtaining a free and well-informed consent from patients before their inclusion in a study. Where possible, a new drug should always first be compared to a placebo in order to prove its superiority. Else, a small-sized trial comparing a new drug versus a reference treatment can lead to an erroneous conclusion of absence of difference. Moreover, good results or improvement are obtained in at least 30% of cases with a placebo, whatever the

---

*Reviewer at the French Drug Agency, member of a Parisian Ethics Committee.

Pharmaceutical Ethics. Edited by S. Salek and A. Edgar.

disease. The use of a placebo is unethical in life-threatening diseases and when an effective proved drug exists. The use of a placebo is ethical in severe diseases with no efficient drug, in some severe diseases even when an efficient standard treatment is available, and in all moderate and functional diseases. In order to detect flawed studies, most journals now ask for any manuscript submitted and reporting results of a randomized clinical trial to join a checklist in order to verify the quality of the trial. Finally, it remains the responsibility of the doctor to decide whether or not a protocol is ethical, to participate or not, and to include patients or not. Everyone has to remember that the interests of the patient must always prevail over the interests of science or society.

Keywords: Ethics committee; Informed consent; Placebo; Publication ethics; Randomized controlled trials; Research ethics

A SHORT HISTORY

One of the first international reflections concerning ethics in human biomedical research was carried out after the 1945 Nuremberg Judgement, where Nazi doctors were prosecuted for their experiments on death camp prisoners. This resulted in the Nuremberg Code (1947–1949), which stated that "human experimentation is ethical only if it leads to benefits for the whole community which cannot be obtained by other means and that several fundamental principles are respected", such as informed consent, the qualification of investigators, or the strict control of the risks for the patients included (1,2). The code already underlined the requisite quality of the methodology and the design of trials. The basic ethical principles of human experimentation were also stated in the Belmont Report in 1979 (3). The current reference guideline is the Declaration of Helsinki (2) of human rights in medical research, published by the World Medical Association in 1964, and revised several times (4a,b). Guidelines were also published by the World Health Organization and the Council of International Organizations of Medical Sciences (5). Whatever the guidelines, three major principles are emphasized: respect, i.e. autonomy of the person to accept or not to participate in a trial; beneficence, i.e. the constraints and the presumed risks must be acceptable for patients included in a study (risk/benefit ratio); justice, i.e. some vulnerable subjects should not participate in studies, unless under strict conditions to protect them.

After the dramatic side-effects of thalidomide involving 20,000 patients, a drug surveillance was developed in the USA, and after a major survey on protection of human subjects in biomedical research, the USA published guidelines on Good Clinical Practice (1974–1978). In 1981, it was strictly compulsory in the USA to obtain the approval of an Institutional Review Board (Ethics Committee) and informed consent from patients before initiating a study. In France, Good Clinical Practice guidelines were published in 1987 and the ethical law for biomedical research ("loi Huriet") in 1988. In 1990 the Good Clinical Practice for trials on medicinal products in the European Community was released, and a European convention on human rights in biomedical research is under completion (6). Finally, through the International Conference on Harmonization (ICH), the European Union, United States and Japan adopted recently the note for guidance on Good Clinical Practice (7).

The principle of justice has not always been respected in the past. The American government recently apologized to survivors of a study on the natural course of syphilis untreated in black men in Tuskegee, AL. 412 poor African–American men were followed from 1932 to 1972, even after penicillin was proved to be highly effective in syphilis and became available (8). These men were not told they had syphilis, and they were not given counselling on avoiding spread of the disease. This is the perfect representation of the potential for exploitation of any population that may be vulnerable because of race, ethnicity, gender, disability, age or social class (8). In 1991, a study on a new hepatitis A vaccine was conducted with Indians in a Sioux reservation. The consent form implied an established prevention programme rather than the safety and efficacy trial of a new vaccine (9).

All the guidelines concerning ethics in biomedical research in Europe or the USA are more or less similar and demand: adherence to the principles of the Declaration of Helsinki, approval of the trial by an Ethics Committee, obtaining of informed consent from patients and compliance with Good Clinical Practice guidelines. These latter include: obligations of sponsors, obligations of clinical investigators, guidelines in case of a serious adverse event, necessity for quality control procedures of the study (monitoring, audit) and strict conditions for performing a trial in vulnerable subjects, especially trials without direct individual benefit. For example, such trials cannot be carried out in children, except if there is absence of foreseeable risk, it is useful for other children of the same age and condition, and it is impossible to conduct it in any other way. The consent of both the parents and the child (if possible) must be obtained. These restrictions are identical for pregnant, parturient, or breast-feeding women, psychomotor impaired adults protected by the law, etc. Table 6.1 presents some of the obligations of the French ethical law. These obligations are even more strict for trials without direct individual benefit, in order to prevent healthy volunteers from frequent involvement in these studies.

The reflection concerning ethics in human research also made it possible to recognize the absolute necessity of conducting clinical trials to prove the efficacy of drugs and their legality. Not so long ago, the French National

Table 6.1   French ethical law "Huriet": presentation of some of the obligations

- Requisite animal studies
- Approval from an ethics committee
- Free and well-informed consent (oral and written)
- Restrictions on participation of vulnerable subjects
- Possibility for patients to stop their participation at any time
- Obligation of an insurance for damage (sponsor)
- Qualification and experience (investigator)
- Dispensation of drugs by pharmacy (applicable for a trial conducted in hospital)
- Drugs, consultations and tests free for the patient when necessitated by the study and not by normal medical care

Trial without direct individual benefit:
- Trial must be performed in an authorized centre
- Inscription of the volunteers on a national file register
- Volunteers must be covered by social security
- Exclusion period during which a subject cannot be included in another trial
- Maximal annual indemnities received by a volunteer (about 3800 Euro per year)
- Liability insurance for the sponsor even if not related directly to the study

Ethics Committees stated (1984) that "It is contrary to ethics to generalise a medical treatment before its efficacy and tolerance have been tested according to a strict method", and the French medical code of professional ethics declared (1988): "Medicine is inevitably experimental".

The efficacy of drugs has to be assessed by clinical trials. But a trial can be unethical if its scientific and methodological quality is poor, such as for example: trial not comparative, not randomized, or without blind procedure (even though it is feasible), no calculation of the number of patients to be included, trial not in compliance with Good Clinical Practice, or flawed analysis strategy (e.g. "per protocol" analysis instead of "intent to treat analysis") (10). The French National Ethics Committees reaffirmed in 1986: "What is not scientific is not ethical".

INFORMED CONSENT

The investigator is responsible for obtaining free and well-informed consent from patients before their inclusion in a study. However, it is often both difficult and lengthy to obtain informed consent from patients (11,12). Explanations regarding trial methodology, especially the randomization, are often barely understood by the patients (13,14) and can result in refusal (15). It is our very personal point of view that this explanation has to be toned down in some patients or circumstances, or the investigator must be prepared to find appropriate and simple words to explain what is a placebo-controlled, randomized, double-blind trial and why it is necessary. In contrast, the following information has to be given to patients: expected benefits (if any), possible risks and adverse events (those frequent and those rare but severe), constraints and discomforts (e.g. number of consultations, number of blood punctures, virological tests such as HIV, genetic test, description of painful or unpleasant tests, length of participation, etc.).

Guidelines do not resolve all the situations. Is the consent really free and well-informed, in patients who are old, hospitalized and confined to bed or suffer from cognitive deficiency (16), or those who live in residential homes and are dependent on the medical and nursing staff? In these borderline cases, the responsibility remains with the investigator to participate and include patients only in useful and well-conceived studies.

In emergency conditions, when it is impossible to ask a patient for consent, e.g. patient with acute thoracic pain or airflow obstruction, informed consent must be asked by proxy (if any), and the deferred informed consent of the patient must be confirmed afterwards (by which time the trial is often over) (17–19). Even strict guidelines allow for the inclusion of patients under such emergency conditions. It would otherwise have been impossible to prove the efficacy of early administration of thrombolytics for acute myocardial infarction (20).

The explanation of placebo is difficult, with the risks of lack of understanding, and refusal. Many Phase III trials fail to obtain a written informed consent because of the placebo (21,22). We do not know how a patient's behaviour is modified by telling him that he has a 50% chance of receiving a placebo. The objective of a trial versus placebo is precisely to evaluate the true effect of the new treatment against a placebo in patients who are unaware of their treatment allocation. In order to help the investigators, the placebo could be presented as follows in oral and written information, without being unethical: *"Substance with no direct effect, but susceptible to contribute to the improvement of the disease"*, *"Half of patients will receive active treatment and the other half a treatment devoid of active substance"*, *"You will receive either active treatment or a treatment without specific activity"*, *"The objective of the study is to compare the effects of 2 treatments containing or not an active substance"*.

It is evident that patients are unlikely to understand all the information which is given to them by whatever means during consent consultations (14). Not only do the rather abstract terms of methodology (controlled trial, randomization, double-blind) raise problems of comprehension (13), but the recall of information about the risk/benefit ratio of treatment options and prognosis (e.g. in cancer) is also limited even in the short term (23,24). Informed consent based on verbal information alone is clearly not enough (23). Moreover, information letters need to be improved. A review of a sample of 101 clinical trial protocols approved in two Spanish university general hospitals showed that the written form of information provided to the patient had serious deficiencies, either in their formal readability or in the amount and quality of the information (25).

The optimal amount of information to be given to patients is debated. Montgomery and Sneyd (26) sent a postal questionnaire to 204 patients who had taken part in clinical trials. The conclusion was that increasing the amount and complexity of information does not alter patient satisfaction. A study tested the hypothesis that a simplified consent form would be less intimidating and more easily understood by individuals with low-to-marginal reading skills (183 adults). Nearly all participants thought that the simplified form was easier to read. However, the degree to which participants understood the forms was similar for the standard and the simplified consent forms, raising concerns about the adequacy of the design of written informed consent documents for such participants (27). Edwards et al. (28) reviewed research reports which provided data on methods of obtaining informed consent. Their results suggest that there is an optimal amount of information which enhances patient understanding and which might, in turn, reduce anxiety. But giving people more information and more time to reflect tends to be associated with a lower consent rate.

Efforts are currently being made to improve the effectiveness and quality of informed consent (29), e.g. development of a model consent document in cancer clinical trials with relevant and understandable information (30), implication of non-physician personnel in the informed consent process, such as nurses (31). Jimison et al. (32) adapted a structured multimedia informed consent system for clinical trials involving patients with potential cognitive impairment (depression, breast cancer, schizophrenia). Nevertheless, the provision of clear and accurate patient information is important, but this alone will not ensure consistent interpretation of concepts such as randomization (13). A high level of reading skill and comprehension is still necessary to understand and complete most consent forms that are required for participation in clinical research studies (27). And fully informed consent for all patients is an unobtainable ideal (14).

Whatever the difficulties, not to correctly inform a patient is not only unethical (33), it is the best way of increasing the risks of patients withdrawing or being lost to follow-up, which can be detrimental to the results of the trial. The simpler the protocol, the fewer the constraints and the more effective the drug, the easier it will be to obtain the informed consent.

Subjects must also be informed about their right to strict confidentiality of their data collected during a clinical trial, which can only be reviewed by investigators, sponsors or regulatory authorities. This is particularly true for the genetic information collected during clinical trials.

ETHICS COMMITTEES

Ethics committees review the protocols submitted and examine in particular the pertinence of the research and appropriateness of the methodology and also try to estimate the ratio between risks and constraints/benefits. Modifications in the protocols are often requested, even those written by large pharmaceuticals companies. These modifications concern mostly the patient information sheet and consent form: difficult to read and understand, too long or too short, omissions (unpleasant test, insurance, etc.), inaccuracies, erroneous translation, spelling mistakes, word processing errors, "cut-copy", etc. (34).

Ethics committees have limitations, as there can be a lack of experts, methodologists or biostatisticians to assess the scientific quality of a very specialized trial, or the methodological quality of a trial (35). One question also often raised is whether a trial is with or without direct individual benefit for participating patients.

A protocol was recently submitted to a local ethics committee in Paris. The objective was to verify the efficacy of an old marketed drug for benign prostatic hyperplasia in an international multicentre, double-blind, randomized trial, versus placebo. 360 patients treated over one year were needed to show that the drug was superior to placebo by a 2.5 points difference on a clinical score ranging from 0 to 35. What is the clinical significance of such a difference? The local ethics committee overlooked this question, although the protocol had been reviewed by an expert in urology.

Some authors propose recommendations for improving the efficacy of ethics committees, such as requiring systematic reviews of existing research before approving a trial, requiring that a summary of relevant systematic reviews be made available to potential participants, requiring registration of clinical trials at inception as a condition of approval, requiring a commitment by investigators to make the results publicly accessible as a condition of approval, and auditing the reporting of results of research previously approved by ethics committees. Unfortunately, these demand trained and skilled people as well as adequate means and money (35). However, Denmark is shortly going to require applicants for ethical approval to show that they have carried out a full systematic review of the relevant scientific literature before the study will be approved (36). And in some countries, like the United States, ethics committees have also the mission of monitoring the progress of studies.

To compensate for these limitations, in certain countries a committee is responsible for re-examining some of the planned trials or trials in progress after the ethics committees (in France: Biomedical Research Group of the French Drug Agency). This committee can reassess the scientific quality of a trial, convert a trial with direct benefit to a trial without direct individual benefit, or re-evaluate the risks/benefit ratio in the light of declared severe adverse events.

IS THE USE OF A PLACEBO IN CLINICAL TRIALS ETHICAL?

For some authors, "placebo is unethical when an active treatment exists" (37–39). Rothman and Michels (40) suggest that the results of previous research in, for example, rheumatoid arthritis, depression, emesis and hypertension, make the use of placebos unethical in recent trials. But then a small-sized trial comparing a new drug versus a reference treatment can lead to an erroneous conclusion of absence of difference or even of equivalence, although there can be a genuine inferiority of the new drug compared to the reference treatment. The comparator treatment may also be a poor drug (37). These can lead to the registration of a less effective drug (41,42). If the treatment is ineffective, a placebo-controlled trial may minimize the number of patients ultimately exposed to an ineffective treatment (43a,b). For many years physicians had treated patients with anti-arrhythmic drugs in an effort to reduce mortality after myocardial infarction, until a placebo-controlled trial revealed that these drugs were increasing mortality (44a). So where possible, a new drug should always first be compared to a placebo in order to prove its superiority before comparing it to other treatments. The question is to decide under which circumstances it becomes unethical to use a placebo.

How many insufficiently powered trials have compared new drugs to reference treatments leading inherently to an absence of difference. Let us imagine a trial comparing a new antidepressant drug to a reference treatment (e.g. clomipramine) in 40 patients. The results are respectively 47% of improvement versus 55%. Due to the small size of the study, the conclusion can only be that there is no difference between the two treatments. Yet, the new drug is inferior to the reference. It may be possible that even in a larger group of patients, comparing the new drug to a placebo would also result in a non-statistical difference, for example 43% versus 40%, the difference in favour of the new drug being not even clinically significant. The final conclusion could be that the new drug is not different from the placebo. There is an ethical choice to be made in the case of a new antidepressant drug: whether to include a few hundred non-suicidal patients in well-conceived and supervised placebo-controlled trials or to accept the risk of a worthless drug (44b,c). Then hundreds of thousands of patients would unknowingly receive an ineffective drug, some for long periods and some while they were suicidal. Would that be ethical (45)? In the case of fluoxetine, of the 14 efficacy studies conducted before the FDA approved the use of fluoxetine, only five showed fluoxetine to be statistically superior to placebo (46). If fluoxetine had not been compared to placebo, it would have been described as being very efficient. A meta-analysis concludes a "relatively modest overall effect size" (47).

When Drug Approval is Based on Weak Data

Interferon is approved in the treatment of chronic viral hepatitis C. Approval was given on the basis of results from small-sized clinical trials. Interferon was associated with a 50% rate of normalization of transaminases at the end of treatment. In fact, relapse is so frequent that now the true remission (disappearance of HCV RNA from serum) rate is believed to be 10 to 15% or even less one year after the end of treatment (48). Compared to this low efficacy, patients are treated for 6 to 12 months, and many experience flu-like symptoms every two days and other side-effects, some of them severe such as depression. Since interferon is registered, it seems unethical for a new antiviral drug to be compared to placebo or to a control group. We believe that it is unethical to expose patients to such an expensive, poorly tolerated and weakly efficient drug over 12 months. In France, heparins were approved for the prevention of deep vein thrombosis in a medical setting, although their efficacy has not been proved (49). Thus, it was judged unethical to conduct trials to prove preventive efficacy versus placebo. Recently, this official approval was removed, and it is once again ethical to compare low molecular weight heparin to a placebo.

Moreover, good results or improvement are obtained in at least 30% of cases with a placebo, whatever the disease (50–65) (Table 6.2). The placebo effect is not solely due to the placebo drug itself (66), but also to the personality of patients and the doctor–patient relationship (67–69), the spontaneous remission of the disease (67,68), the number of consultations in the trial (60), the concurrent medications and regimens and the routine medical and nursing care (68,69), the patients' expectancies regarding the effect of the drug, the quality and the type of information (positive or negative) they receive, the belief and verbal attitudes of the investigators (70–72b), and so on. So even if the patient receives the placebo, he will obtain some benefit most of the time (14). In general, a trial comparing a new drug to a reference treatment results in a higher effect whatever the treatment group, probably because investigators are more confident to inform their patients that they will receive, whatever the treatment allocation, an active treatment. In contrast, a placebo-controlled trial generally leads to a smaller effect whatever the treatment arm, and reflects more accurately the true effect of the drug.

Table 6.2   Placebo effect in different diseases

Disease (reference)	Outcome	Patients (%)
Migraine (52)	Sedation	25
Reflux oesophagitis (53)	Healing after 4 to 8 weeks of treatment	27
Acute nephritic colic (54)	Partial or complete sedation 30 min after the infusion	30
Cancer pain (55)	Short-term improvement in patients suffering from bone metastatic pain or other cancers	30–40
Metastatic prostatic cancer (56)	Partial or complete regression	33
Benign prostatic hyperplasia (57)	Clinical (Boyarski, I-PSS) score or urinary flow rate improvement	30–42
Schizophrenia (58)	Improvement	6–43
Depression (59)	Improvement greater than 50% in Hamilton depression score	30–40
Ulcerative colitis (60)	Clinical benefit	38.5
Duodenal ulcer disease (61)	Healing at 4 weeks	40–50
Irritable bowel syndrome (62)	Pain improvement	45
Gastro-oesophageal reflux disease (63)	Partial or complete resolution of symptoms	9–69
Dyspepsia (64)	Symptom improvement	13–73
Chronic occlusive peripheral arterial disease (65)	Improvement of claudication distance	60

Including a placebo group in a randomized controlled trial changes how patients rate the efficacy and adverse effects of treatments. Rochon et al. reviewed 58 trials evaluating non-steroidal anti-inflammatory drugs (NSAIDs) in arthritis patients (25 trials versus placebo and 33 trials versus active treatment). Patients receiving NSAIDs in a placebo-controlled trial were more likely to withdraw due to inefficacy, but withdrawals due to adverse events were found to be more common when the NSAIDs were given in trials that did not include a placebo group (73).

The use of a placebo is certainly unethical in life-threatening diseases (and in diseases for which not treating for the duration of the study might result in irreversible morbidity), and when an effective proved drug exists, like a severe infectious disease, myocardial infarction, pulmonary embolism (unless all patients receive an efficient treatment and a new drug or its placebo) (37–40,74). The use of a placebo is ethical in severe diseases with no efficient drug—a difference has to be made between an established but untested drug and a well-evaluated and efficient drug—in some severe diseases even when an efficient standard treatment is available and when there is no irreversible morbidity of placebo treatment for the duration of the study (58,74–76), and in all moderate and functional diseases. Placebo is especially necessary in situations in which placebo response rates are high, variable or close to response rates for effective therapies (75).

Protocols must contain guarantees to protect patients, especially when the trial is placebo-controlled by exposing patients to placebo for the least amount of time and with possible withdrawal of patients after a few weeks of treatment in the event of inefficiency (e.g. depression), possible rescue treatment (especially in painful diseases like migraine), inclusion of moderate cases (like in diabetes or hypertension), and no inclusion of major concomitant risk factors (e.g. cardiovascular) (76,77). Thus, the criteria of "non-response" of patients to therapy should be clearly defined in the protocol (at what delay? which end-point level?) (78).

The methodology and the safety of short-term placebo-controlled trials are well documented in many diseases, such as cardiovascular diseases (systemic hypertension, angina pectoris, chronic heart failure, ventricular tachyarrhythmias) (76,77). In any case, patients included in a trial and even those receiving placebo are better followed than in a normal medical setting, since they are examined and monitored at several consultations and receive the regular advice of a physician.

The issues become more complex with long-term studies in some chronic conditions. For example, a long-term trial with a placebo control in mild hypertension may appear unethical because untreated patients are at an increased risk of morbidity and mortality. In these situations, the decision to include or not a placebo group in a clinical trial in order to assess the efficacy of a new drug should depend upon the severity of the disease, the rate at which the disease may cause irreversible damage, and the availability of an effective treatment (78).

In summary, the randomized controlled trial versus placebo, by subtracting the amount of placebo effect, allows us to determine the presence or not of specific drug effects and may prevent the use of ineffective or dangerous treatments (68,78). Placebo control is appropriate in conditions for which equipoise applies, i.e. the risk/benefit ratios of the different arms of a study are uncertain (68,78,79).

ETHICS AND INTERNATIONAL RESEARCH

Research standards are the same throughout the world, but medical care is not (80). Study ACTG 076 conducted in the USA and France showed that a complex regimen of zidovudine reduced the incidence of maternal–infant HIV transmission from 25.5% (placebo) to 8.3% (81). This ACTG 076 regimen was then recommended for all HIV-positive pregnant women in developed countries. But after the results of the trial, several studies in developing countries compared a shorter regimen—less expensive—to placebo. The question raised by several authors is: should an effective treatment for which new studies versus placebo would be unethical in developed countries, be ethical in developing countries (82)?

The arguments for such placebo-controlled trials in developing countries are somewhat weak (80): American and African populations are different, so one does not know if the ACTG 076 complex regimen is active in Africa. African women would in any case never receive such an expensive regimen, and if a shorter regimen proved to be superior to the placebo, it would serve only developing countries. This latter argument is false. It is clear that if such a shorter regimen was effective, it would also be used in developed countries. So, the use of placebo in this case seems unethical. The ethical study to be performed could be a trial comparing a complex regimen to a shorter regimen of zidovudine (82). Differences in healthcare needs and budgets should not justify different ethical standards in the developed and the developing world (83).

It is debated whether it is possible to have one internationally recognized standard of "informed consent" or whether research ethics should be adapted to the culture and educational level of the study population. Leach et al. (84) examined the attitudes of the Gambian people to consent to medical research, and evaluated the informed consent process used in a trial of a *Haemophilus influenzae* vaccine. Except for the placebo control design, which was understood by only 10% of participants, other points of knowledge were well recalled. Therefore, at least in Gambia, the international code of informed consent is appropriate.

PUBLICATIONS

It is unethical to publish flawed studies and not to publish negative studies (85). In order to increase the quality of manuscripts, most journals now ask for any manuscript submitted and reporting results of a randomized clinical trial to join a checklist (CONSORT) in order to verify the quality of the trial (86–88). But even major journals published, until the recent past, poorly designed trials or flawed analyses. In a trial comparing octreotide infusion to sclerotherapy for variceal haemorrhage and published in 1993 by *The Lancet*, the authors explained their hypotheses in the statistical methods section: "Based on an expected efficacy of 85% with octreotide and 90% with sclerotherapy, and a two-tailed test, alpha error 5%, beta error 20%, we estimated at least 900 patients in each group were needed . . . We arbitrarily set a target of 100 patients and accepted a chance of type II error (β)". As for results, the authors effectively included 100 patients. Bleeding was controlled in 84% with octreotide and 90% with sclerotherapy. Unsurprisingly there was no significant difference ($p = 0.55$). The conclusion was misinterpreted: "We conclude that octreotide infusion and emergency sclerotherapy are equally effective in controlling variceal haemorrhage" (89). Other flawed analyses concern: lack of comparability between treatment groups at randomization, mostly due to the low number of subjects included (90); high number of patients lost to follow-up or per protocol analysis, thus excluding many patients from analysis (91–94b); intra-group comparison without comparison between treatment groups (93,94); subgroup analysis without stratification (91).

The presentation of results can also be rather unethical (95). Results expressed as relative risk reduction should be avoided. Misoprostol reduces by 51% (relative risk reduction) serious gastrointestinal events in patients receiving NSAIDs, compared to placebo (96). This reduction is statistically significant and sounds clinically pertinent. But, the absolute risk reduction is only 3.8% (percentage of events: placebo 7.4%, misoprostol 3.6%). Much more informative is the number of patients needed to treat (reciprocal of the absolute risk reduction) (97): 263 patients are needed to be treated by misoprostol over 6 months to avoid one case of serious gastrointestinal event. At the same time, for every 13 patients treated, one patient will experience diarrhoea or abdominal pain severe enough to stop the drug. This number gives a more accurate reflection of the clinical pertinence of the benefit of the drug. Another example exerts the same relative risk reduction but a much lower number of patients needed to treat, just because the occurrence of an event is higher (98). Anticoagulant therapy reduces by 53% compared to placebo the risk of recurrence of stroke in patients with atrial fibrillation. Absolute risk reduction is 9% (percentage of events: placebo 17%, anticoagulant 8%). Thus, only 11 patients treated for one year are needed to avoid one case of recurrence of stroke. So results should present not only absolute numbers and the value of p, but also the confidence interval ($CI_{95\%}$) (99) and the number of patients needed to treat (97).

Moreover, any conflict of interest or financial relationship between pharmaceutical companies and authors of papers reporting trial results should be disclosed.

ADVERTISING

International guidelines on ethics, on good clinical practice and more recently on publications are accepted and adhered to throughout the world. Such guidelines should also be followed for advertisements and promotional documents (100). Many of these documents are flawed in that they omit data (e.g. selecting only the studies in favour of the treatment), use superlative adjectives, present scientific data derived from animals and not supported by any clinical data, or suggest the use of the drug in indications which are not approved (Tables 6.3 and 6.4). The marketing information

Table 6.3 Unethical promotional document with H_2-receptor antagonist: percentage of duodenal ulcer healing at 4 weeks[a]

Author (year)	Classen (1985)	Mulder (1989)	Hui (1989)	Sabbatini (1988)
H_2-receptor antagonist	92	96	93	91
Proton pump inhibitor	96	91	96	92

[a] Truncated information by presenting four selected studies favouring the treatment (that is no statistical difference between the H_2-receptor antagonist and a proton pump inhibitor). The true healing percentage is nearer to 80% for this H_2-receptor antagonist and 95% for the proton pump inhibitor (61).

Table 6.4 Unethical promotional document on a "hepatic protector"

1. Drug X inhibits lipidic peroxidation, increases membrane stabilization and enzymatic stimulation[a]
2. Drug X protects the liver from aggressions (virus, alcohol, drugs, etc.)[b]
3. Drug X will make hepatic disorders (fatigue, dyspepsia, anorexia, etc.) disappear[b]
4. To help your patients to recover a normal hepatic function[b]
5. You will see the difference objectively

[a] Document uses superlative adjectives and indications not approved. The only bibliographic references are old, reporting only results in vitro or in rats.
[b] This assertion is not based on any clinical trial.

delivered by pharmaceutical companies to clinicians and pharmacists raises a real ethical question, particularly since the development of new media like the web or internet (101). Advertising concerns also new outcome criteria such as quality of life, whose results are still difficult to interpret for clinicians. Although the need to assess subjective aspects of health-related quality of life under chronic conditions is now increasingly recognized (102,103), the analysis and presentation of results of quality of life data in clinical trials is often flawed (104). Thus reporting on quality of life in clinical trials should be significantly improved and should follow the CONSORT guidelines like any clinical trial (105).

FRAUD STILL EXISTS

Falsification and fabrication of data still exist in spite of the fact that investigators are aware that their work can be controlled by monitoring and possible audit (106). A well-known example is the fraud committed by an academic from Montreal during several breast-cancer trials (107). Forged consent forms from patients and forged ethics committee approvals are also revealed (108). Since 1977, the FDA has conducted 4154 inspections of trials:

53% of investigators clearly failed to disclose the experimental nature of their work. In 46 trials, drugs were tested without any written evidence that subjects had consented (9). Other unethical behaviour concerns plagiarism, or insider dealing.

CONCLUSION

At the basis, there is the relationship between a patient and a doctor. Finally, it remains the responsibility of the doctor to decide whether or not a protocol is ethical, to participate or not, and to include patients or not: are the objectives pertinent and useful for patients? Is the methodology correct? Is the risk/benefit ratio acceptable for patients? Everyone has to remember that the interests of the patient must always prevail over the interests of science or society.

REFERENCES

1. Shuster E. Fifty years later: the significance of the Nuremberg Code. *N Engl J Med* 1997; **337**: 1436–40.
2. The Nuremberg Code (1947). Declaration of Helsinki (1964). *BMJ* 1996; **313**: 1448–9.
3. Belmont report. Web site: http://ohrp.osophs.dhhs.gov/humansubjects/guidance/belmont.htm
4. (a) World Medical Association Declaration of Helsinki. Recommendations guiding physicians in biomedical research involving human subjects. *JAMA* 1997; **277**: 925–6. (b) Ethical Principles for Medical Research Involving Human Subjects. Updated at the 52nd World Medical Association General Assembly, Edinburgh, Scotland, October 2000. *Bull World Health Org* 2001; **79**: 373–4.
5. CIOMS/WHO. *International Ethical Guidelines for Biomedical Research Involving Humans Subjects.* Geneva: CIOMS, 1993.
6. Convention pour la protection des droits de l'homme et de la dignité de l'être humain à l'égard des applications de la biologie et de la médecine: convention sur les droits de l'homme et la biomédecine. Council of Europe, Strasbourg, November 1996.
7. Note for guidance on good clinical practice. The European Agency for the Evaluation of Medicinal Products. CPMP/ICH/135/95. Web site: http://www.eudra.org/humandocs/PDFs/ICH/013595en.pdf
8. Corbie-Smith G. The continuing legacy of the Tuskegee Syphilis Study: considerations for clinical investigation. *Am J Med Sci* 1999; **317**: 5–8.
9. Epstein K, Sloat B. Informed consent is not always obtained in United States. *BMJ* 1997; **315**: 247.

10. Pfeffer N, Alderson P. The central problem is often poor design and conduct of trials. *BMJ* 1997; **315**: 247.
11. Wager E, Tooley PJH, Emanuel MB, Wood SF. Get patient's consent to enter clinical trials. *BMJ* 1995; **311**: 734–7.
12. Riordan FAI, Thompson APJ. How to get patients' consent to enter clinical trials. *BMJ* 1996; **312**: 185–6.
13. Featherstone K, Donovan JL. Random allocation or allocation at random? Patients' perspectives of participation in a randomised controlled trial. *BMJ* 1998; **317**: 1177–80.
14. Edwards SJ, Lilford RJ, Braunholtz DA, Jackson JC, Hewison J, Thornton J. Ethical issues in the design and conduct of randomised controlled trials. *Health Technol Assess* 1998; **2**: 1–132.
15. Elbourne D, Snowdon C, Garcia J. Subjects may not understand concept of clinical trials. *BMJ* 1997; **315**: 247.
16. High DM. Research with Alzheimer's disease subjects: informed consent and proxy decision making. *J Am Geriatr Soc* 1992; **40**: 950–7.
17. Morley C. Consent is not always practical in emergency treatments. *BMJ* 1997; **314**: 1480.
18. Slyter H. Ethical challenges in stroke research. *Stroke* 1998; **29**: 1725–9.
19. Clement S. Full information about trials might be given retrospectively to participants. *BMJ* 1999; **318**: 736.
20. Ketley D, Woods KL. Impact of clinical trials on clinical practice: example of thrombolysis for acute myocardial infarction. *Lancet* 1993; **342**: 891–4.
21. Adedeji OA. Informed consent in clinical trials. *BMJ* 1993; **307**: 1494–7.
22. Waldrom HA, Cookson RF. Avoiding the pitfalls of sponsored multicentre research in general practice. *BMJ* 1993; **307**: 1331–4.
23. Lloyd AJ, Hayes PD, London NJM, Bell PRF, Naylor AR. Patients' ability to recall risk associated with treatment options. *Lancet* 1999; **353**: 645–6.
24. Gattelari M, Butow PN, Tattersall MHN. Informed consent: what did the doctor say? *Lancet* 1999; **353**: 1713.
25. Ordovas Baines JP, Lopez Briz E, Urbieta Sanz E, Torregrosa Sanchez R, Jimenez Torres NV. An analysis of patient information sheets for obtaining informed consent in clinical trials. *Med Clin (Barc)* 1999; **112**: 90–4.
26. Montgomery JE, Sneyd JR. Consent to clinical trials in anaesthesia. *Anaesthesia* 1998; **53**: 227–30.
27. Davis TC, Holcombe RF, Berkel HJ, Pramanik S, Divers SG. Informed consent for clinical trials: a comparative study of standard versus simplified forms. *J Natl Cancer Inst* 1998; **90**: 668–74.
28. Edwards SJ, Lilford RJ, Thornton J, Hewison J. Informed consent for clinical trials: in search of the "best" method. *Soc Sci Med* 1998; **47**: 1825–40.
29. Lavori PW, Sugarman J, Hays MT, Feussner JR. Improving informed consent in clinical trials: a duty to experiment. *Control Clin Trials* 1999; **20**: 187–93.
30. Padberg RM, Flach J. National efforts to improve the informed consent process. *Semin Oncol Nurs* 1999; **15**: 138–44.
31. McCabe MS. The ethical foundation of informed consent in clinical research. *Semin Oncol Nurs* 1999; **15**: 76–80.
32. Jimison HB, Sher PP, Appleyard R, LeVernois Y. The use of multimedia in the informed consent process. *J Am Med Inform Assoc* 1998; **5**: 245–56.
33. Sikorski J. Lack of respect for patients in medical research may reflect wider disrespect in clinical practice. *BMJ* 1997; **315**: 250.

34. Priestley K, Campbell C, Valentine C, Denison D, Buller N. Are patient consent forms for research protocols easy to read? *BMJ* 1992; **305**: 1263–4.
35. Blunt J, Savulescu J, Watson AJM. Meeting the challenges facing research ethics committees: some practical suggestions. *BMJ* 1998; **316**: 58–61.
36. Goldbeck-Wood S. Denmark takes a lead on research ethics. *BMJ* 1998; **316**: 1185.
37. Henry D, Hill S. Comparing treatments. Comparison should be against active treatments rather than placebo. *BMJ* 1995; **310**: 1279.
38. Brody BA. When are placebo-controlled trials no longer appropriate? *Control Clin Trials* 1997; **18**: 602–12.
39. Simon R. Are placebo-controlled clinical trials ethical or needed when alternative treatment exists? *Ann Intern Med* 2000; **133**: 474–5.
40. Rothman KJ, Michels KB. Declaration of Helsinki should be strengthened. *BMJ* 2000; **321**: 442–4.
41. Greene WL, Concato J, Feinstein AR. Claims of equivalence in medical research: are they supported by the evidence? *Ann Intern Med* 2000; **132**: 715–22.
42. Jones B, Jarvis P, Lewis JA, Ebbutt AF. Trials to assess equivalence: the importance of rigorous methods. *BMJ* 1996; **313**; 36–9.
43. (a) Temple R, Ellenberg SS. Placebo-controlled trials and active-control trials in the evaluation of new treatments. Part 1: Ethical and scientific issues. *Ann Intern Med* 2000; **133**: 455–63. (b) Leon AC. Can placebo controls reduce the number of non responders in clinical trials? A power-analytic perspective. *Clin Ther* 2001; **23**: 596–603.
44. (a) Echt DS, Liebson PB, Mitchell LB, Peters RW, Obias-Manno D, Barker AH et al. Mortality and morbidity in patients receiving encainide, flecainide, or placebo: the cardiac arrhythmia suppression trial. *N Engl J Med* 1991; **324**: 781–8. (b) Khan A, Warner HA, Brown WA. Symptom reduction and suicide risk in patients treated with placebo in antidepressant clinical trials: an analysis of the Food and Drug Administration database. *Arch Gen Psychiatry* 2000; **57**: 311–7. (c) Miller FG. Placebo-controlled trials in psychiatric research: an ethical perspective. *Biol Psychiatry* 2000; **47**: 707–16.
45. Pohl R, Balon R. The use of placebo controls. *N Engl J Med* 1995; **332**: 60.
46. Sramek JJ, Cutler NR. The use of placebo controls. *N Engl J Med* 1995; **332**: 60.
47. Greenberg RP, Bornstein RF, Zborowski MJ, Fisher S, Greenberg MD. A meta-analysis of fluoxetine outcome in the treatment of depression. *J Nerv Ment Dis* 1994; **182**: 547–51.
48. Chassany O. Treatment of viral hepatitis C. *Presse Med* 1996; **25**: 1945–51.
49. Bergmann JF, Caulin C. Heparin prophylaxis in bedridden patients. *Lancet* 1996; **348**: 205–6.
50. Bostrom H. Placebo—the forgotten drug. *Scand J Work Environ Health* 1997; **23** (Suppl 3): 53–7.
51. Ernst E, Herxheimer A. The power of placebo. *BMJ* 1996; **313**: 1569–70.
52. Tfelt-Hansen P, Henry P, Mulder LJ, Scheldewaert RG, Schoenen J, Chazot G. The effectiveness of combined lysine acetylsalicylate and metoclopramide compared with sumatriptan for migraine. *Lancet* 1995; **346**: 923–6.
53. Pace F, Maconi G, Molteni P, Minguzzi M, Bianchi Porro G. Meta-analysis of the effect of placebo on the outcome of medically treated reflux esophagitis. *Scand J Gastroenterol* 1995; **30**: 101–5.
54. Holmhund D, Sjödin JG. Treatment of ureteral colic with intra-venous indomethacin. *J Urol* 1978; **120**: 676–7.

55. Boureau F, Leizorovicz A, Caulin F. The placebo effect in bone metastatic pain. *Presse Med* 1988; **17**: 1063–6.
56. Bertagna C, De Géry A, Hucher M, François JP, Zanirato J. Efficacy of the combination of nilutamide plus orchidectomy in patients with metastatic prostatic cancer. A meta-analysis of seven randomized double-blind trials (1056 patients). *Br J Urol* 1994; **73**: 396–402.
57. Isaacs JT. Importance of natural history of benign prostatic hyperplasia in the evaluation of pharmacologic intervention. *Prostate* 1990; **3** (Suppl): S1–7.
58. Storosum JG, Elferink AJ, Van Zwieen BJ. Schizophrenia: do we really need placebo-controlled studies? *Eur Neuropsychopharmacol* 1998; **8**: 279–86.
59. Brown WA, Dornseif BE, Wernicke JF. Placebo response in depression: a search for predictors. *Psychiatry Res* 1988; **26**: 259–64.
60. Ilnyckyj A, Shanahan F, Anton PA, Cheang M, Bernstein CN. Quantification of the placebo response in ulcerative colitis. *Gastroenterology* 1997; **112**: 1854–8.
61. Anti-ulcer agents. Recommandations and medical references. Agence Nationale pour le Développement de l'Évaluation Médicale (ANDEM). *Gastroenterol Clin Biol* 1996; **20**: 991–1008.
62. Poynard T, Naveau S, Mory B, Chaput JC. Meta-analysis of smooth relaxants in the treatment of irritable bowel syndrome. *Aliment Pharmacol Ther* 1994; **8**: 499–510.
63. Sontag SJ. Rolling review: gastro-oesophageal reflux disease. *Aliment Pharmacol Ther* 1993; **7**: 293–312.
64. Hansen JM, Bytzer P, Schaffalitzky de Muckadell OB. Placebo-controlled trial of cisapride and nizatidine in unselected patients with functional dyspepsia. *Am J Gastroenterol* 1998; **93**: 368–74.
65. Lindgärde F, Jelnes R, Bjorkman H, Adielsson G, Kjellstrom T, Palmquist I, Stavenow L. Conservative drug treatment in patients with moderately severe chronic occlusive peripheral arterial disease. Scandinavian Study Group. *Circulation* 1989; **80**: 1549–56.
66. De Craen AJ, Roos PJ, Leonard de Vries A, Kleijnen J. Effect of colour of drugs: systematic review of perceived effect of drugs and of their effectiveness. *BMJ* 1996; **313**: 1624–6.
67. Dobrilla G, Scarpignato C. Placebo and placebo effect: their impact on the evaluation of drug response in patients. *Dig Dis* 1994; **12**: 368–77.
68. Kaptchuk TJ. Powerful placebo: the dark side of the randomised controlled trial. *Lancet* 1998; **351**: 1722–5.
69. Kienle GS, Kiene H. Placebo effect and placebo concept: a critical methodological and conceptual analysis of reports on the magnitude of the placebo effect. *Altern Ther* 1996; **2**: 39–54.
70. Bergmann JF, Chassany O, Gandiol J, Deblois P, Kanis JA, Caulin C, Dahan R. A randomised clinical trial of the effect of informed consent on the analgesic activity of placebo and naproxen in cancer pain. *Clin Trials Meta-Anal* 1994; **29**: 41–7.
71. Kleijnen J, De Craen AJM, Van Everdingen J, Krol L. Placebo effects in double-blind clinical trials: a review of interactions with medications. *Lancet* 1994; **344**: 1347–9.
72. (a) Fillmore M, Vogel-Sprott M. Expected effect of caffeine on motor performance predicts the type of response to placebo. *Psychopharmacology* 1992; **106**: 209–14. (b) Flaten MA, Simonsen T, Olsen H. Drug-related information generates placebo and nocebo responses that modify the drug response. *Psychosom Med* 1999; **61**: 250–5.

73. Rochon PA, Binns MA, Litner JA, Litner GM, Fischbach MS, Eisenberg D, Kaptchuk TJ, Stason WB, Chalmers TC. Are randomized control trial outcomes influenced by the inclusion of a placebo group?: a systematic review of non-steroidal antiinflammatory drug trials for arthritis treatment. *J Clin Epidemiol* 1999; **52**: 113–22.

74. Clark PI, Leaverton PE. Scientific and ethical issues in the use of placebo controls in clinical trials. *Ann Rev Public Health* 1994; **15**: 19–38.

75. Addington D, Williams R, Lapierre Y, El-Guebaly N. Placebos in clinical trials of psychotropic medication. *Can J Psychiatry* 1997; **42**:6P.

76. Bienenfeld L, Frishman W, Glasser SP. The placebo effect in cardiovascular disease. *Am Heart J* 1996; **132**: 1207–21.

77. Weber MA. The ethics of using placebo in hypertension clinical trials. *J Hypertens* 1999; **17**: 5–8.

78. Stein CM, Pincus T. Placebo-controlled studies in rheumatoid arthritis: ethical issues. *Lancet* 1999; **353**: 4000–3.

79. Avins AL. Can unequal be more fair? Ethics, subject allocation, and randomised clinical trials. *J Med Ethics* 1998; **24**: 401–8.

80. Halsey NE, Sommer A, Henderson DA, Black RE. Ethics and international research. *BMJ* 1997; **315**: 965–6.

81. Connor EM, Sperling RS, Geiber R, Kiselev P, Scott G, O'Sullivan MJ et al. Reduction of maternal–infant transmission of human immunodeficiency virus type 1 with zidovudine treatment. *N Engl J Med* 1994; **331**: 1173–80.

82. Lurie P, Wolfe SM. Unethical trials of interventions to reduce perinatal transmission of the human immunodeficiency virus in developing countries. *N Engl J Med* 1997; **337**: 853–6.

83. Studdert DM, Brennan TA. Clinical trials in developing countries: scientific and ethical issues. *Med J Aust* 1998; **169**: 545–8.

84. Leach A, Hilton S, Greenwood BM, Manneh E, Dibba B, Wilkins A, Mulholland EK. An evaluation of the informed consent procedure used during a trial of a *Haemophilus influenzae* type B conjugate vaccine undertaken in the Gambia, West Africa. *Soc Sci Med* 1999; **48**: 139–48.

85. Smith R, Roberts I. An amnesty for unpublished trials. *BMJ* 1997; **315**: 622.

86. Moher D, Schulz KF, Altman D, CONSORT Group (Consolidated Standards of Reporting Trials). The CONSORT statement: revised recommendations for improving the quality of reports of parallel-group randomized trials. *JAMA* 2001; **285**: 1987–91.

87. Altman DG, Schulz KF, Moher D, Egger M, Davidoff F, Elbourne D, Gotzsche PC, Lang T, CONSORT GROUP (Consolidated Standards of Reporting Trials). The revised CONSORT statement for reporting randomized trials: explanation and elaboration. *Ann Intern Med* 2001; **134**: 663–94.

88. Cleophas RC, Cleophas TJ. Is selective reporting of clinical research unethical as well as unscientific? *Int J Clin Pharmacol Ther* 1999; **37**: 1–7.

89. Sung JY, Sydney Chung SC, Lai C-W, Chan FKL, Leung JWC, Yung M-Y, Kassianides C, Li AKC. Octreotide infusion or emergency sclerotherapy for variceal haemorrhage. *Lancet* 1993; **342**: 637–41.

90. Noble RE. A six-month study of the effects of dexfenfluramine on partially successful dieters. *Curr Ther Res* 1990; **47**: 612–9.

91. O'Driscoll BR, Taylor RJ, Horsley MG, Chambers DK, Bernstein A. Nebulised salbutamol with and without ipatropium bromide in acute airflow obstruction. *Lancet* 1989; **1** (8652): 1418–20.

92. Guy-Grand B, Apfelbaum M, Crepaldi G, Gries A, Lefebvre P, Turner P. International trial of long-term dexfenfluramine in obesity. *Lancet* 1989; **2** (8672): 1142–5.
93. Spechler SJ, Department of Veterans Affairs Gastroesophageal Reflux Disease Study Group. Comparison of medical and surgical therapy for complicated gastroesophageal reflux disease in veterans. *N Engl J Med* 1992; **326**: 786–92.
94. (a) Chassany O, Bergmann JF, Caulin C. Treatment of gastro-oesophageal reflux disease in adults. Efficacy of surgery needs to be compared with that of proton pump inhibitors. *BMJ* 1999; **318**: 59. (b) Chassany O, Fullerton S. Limitation of meta-analysis in regard to selection of studies and interpretation of results. *Am J Med* 2000; **108**: 596–7.
95. McNamee D, Horton R. Lies, damn lies, and reports of RCTs. *Lancet* 1996; **348**: 562.
96. Silverstein FE, Graham DY, Senior JR, Wyn Davies H, Struthers BJ, Bittman RM, Geis S. Misoprostol reduces serious gastrointestinal complications in patients with rheumatoid arthritis receiving nonsteroidal anti-inflammatory drugs. A randomized, double-blind, placebo-controlled trial. *Ann Intern Med* 1995; **123**: 241–9.
97. Cook RJ, Sackett DL. The number needed to treat: a clinically useful measure of treatment effect. *BMJ* 1995; **310**: 452–4.
98. EAFTG. Secondary prevention in non rheumatic atrial fibrillation after transient ischaemic attack or minor stroke. *Lancet* 1993; **342**: 1255–62.
99. Gardner MJ, Altman DG. Confidence intervals rather than P values: estimation rather than hypothesis testing. *BMJ* 1986; **292**: 746–50.
100. Publicité et bon usage. Recommandations de la commission chargée du contrôle de la publicité et de la diffusion de recommandations sur le bon usage du médicament. Agence du Médicament, June 1995.
101. Kim P, Eng TR, Deering MJ, Maxfield A. Published criteria for evaluating health related web sites: review. *BMJ* 1999; **318**: 647–9.
102. Chassany O, Marquis P, Scherrer B, Read NW, Finger T, Bergmann JF, Fraitag B, Geneve J, Caulin C. Validation of a specific quality of life questionnaire in functional digestive disorders (FDDQL). *Gut* 1999; **44**: 527–33.
103. Bergmann JF, Chassany O. Quality of life in functional gastrointestinal disorders: regulatory issues. *Eur J Surg* 1998; **583** (Suppl): 87–91.
104. Sanders C, Egger M, Donovan J, Tallon D, Frankel S. Reporting on quality of life in randomised controlled trials: bibliographic study. *BMJ* 1998; **317**: 1191–4.
105. Chassany O, Sagnier P, Marquis P, Fullerton S, Aaronson N, for the European Regulatory Issues on Quality of Life Assessment (ERIQA) Group. Patient-reported outcomes: the example of health-related quality of life—a European guidance document for the improved integration of health-related quality of life assessment in the drug approval process. *Drug Inf Assoc J* 2002; **36**: 209–38.
106. Bowie C. Was the paper I wrote a fraud? *BMJ* 1998; **316**: 1755–6.
107. Fischer B, Redmond CK. Fraud in breast-cancer trials. *N Engl J Med* 1994; **330**: 1458.
108. Dyer O. GP struck off for fraud in drug trials. *BMJ* 1996; **312**: 798.

7

Can we Afford the Medicines we Need: An Ethical Dilemma?

ROGER WALKER

Gwent Health Authority, Pontypool, Gwent, UK & Welsh School of Pharmacy,
Cardiff University, Cardiff, UK

People continue to expect ever more from their health service. This, together with continuing advances in technology and medicine, explains in part why health care has the potential to become increasingly more expensive. Monies for the provision of health care are not infinite and in every health care system there is a point where resources are no longer adequate and decisions about competing demands have to be made. This situation is largely inevitable in a state run health care system such as that in the UK, where it is acknowledged that the task of government is not to provide the best health care for the least possible cash but to provide, via taxation, the best possible health care from within a limited budget (1).

This chapter looks at the issues behind the management of expenditure on medicines and highlights some of the dilemmas for those who make purchasing decisions. In particular the link between expenditure on medicines and health gain, whether the increased prescription of medicines is fuelled by need, and the criteria for determining need and setting priorities will all be discussed.

Pharmaceutical Ethics. Edited by S. Salek and A. Edgar.
© 2002 John Wiley & Sons, Ltd.

Pharmaceutical Ethics

EXPENDITURE AND HEALTH GAIN

The increasing cost of providing health care is a concern to governments worldwide. In the UK total health care expenditure reached £63 billion in 2000. However, it is not cost alone that is of concern. There is mounting evidence that increased expenditure does not guarantee readily quantifiable improvements in health. For example, using residual life expectancy as a health indicator in the UK (2), a 65-year-old male in 1948 would have expected to live a further 13 years, whilst in 1996 a male of the same age could expect a further 15 years (Table 7.1). In comparison, the UK health service cost £444 million in 1948 compared to £42 billion in 1996; i.e. a 95-fold increase in cost (four-fold in real terms) purchased an additional two years of life. Similarly, comparison of total health expenditure per person, or percentage of gross domestic product spent on health in member countries of the Organization for Economic Cooperation and Development (OECD) (2) shows little relationship with outcomes such as infant mortality and life expectancy (Table 7.2).

Table 7.1 Residual life expectancy (years) amongst males of different ages in England and Wales in 1948 and 1996

Year	Birth	Age 1	Age 15	Age 65
1948	66	68	55	13
1996	74	74	60	15

Source: Adapted from OHE Compendium of Health Statistics, 10th edn, 1997.

Table 7.2 Comparison of life expectancy with percentage gross domestic product (% GDP) spent on health, expenditure per person on health care, prescriptions per 1000 population and infant death rate (per 1000 live births) in different countries

	% GDP	Expenditure per person (£)	Prescriptions per 1000 population	Infant death rate	Life expectancy (years)
Czech Republic	7.6	172	—[a]	7.9	70
Portugal	7.6	435	21.0	8.1	71
Denmark	6.6	1214	7.1	5.6	72
USA	14.3	2285	—[a]	7.9	72
Belgium	8.2	1199	9.5	7.6	73
Finland	8.3	1041	5.7	4.6	73
France	9.7	1449	52.2	5.8	74
Germany	9.5	1552	11.5	5.6	74
UK	6.9	787	10.0	6.2	74
Italy	8.3	967	5.2	6.6	75
Netherlands	8.8	1245	11.0	5.6	75

[a] Data not available.
Source: Adapted from OHE Compendium of Health Statistics, 10th edn, 1997.

Further comparison across OECD countries also reveals no relationship between the number of prescription items per person and health outcomes. Likewise, although the health service in England is less well funded than in other parts of the UK, there is little evidence that this leads to worse outcomes (3). The explanation for this is complex and probably involves the interrelationship between public health, the social/welfare support available to a given population, the efficient use of resources, and the possession of few indicators sensitive to changing patterns of health. The simple message is that spending more on medicines and health does not readily translate to measurable health gain, and this certainly does not arise in a time frame that gives kudos to the ruling political party.

MEDICINES AND NEED

Despite the reservations discussed above, medicines have undoubtedly helped reduce morbidity and mortality over the past 50 years. In the UK it has been estimated that medicines have contributed to a reduction in the average length of hospital stay from 50 days in 1948 to 8 in 1995. It is clear that the benefits of medicines must be harnessed and the challenge for those managing health care, whatever their health care system, is to develop a robust, efficient, evidence-based process to ensure the technologies and medicines that people need are purchased, whilst ineffective procedures and medicines are discontinued. This appears simple and straightforward but it can easily be lost in the ever-present whirlwind of political change that exists in state run health care systems. For example, it is arguable that the emphasis in recent years on delivering ever more efficient health care in the UK has been at the expense of ensuring equity in service access. This is now being addressed, but the issue of "what is need" remains largely unresolved.

Demand is often considered as a "want" and/or a "need". Some needs are wants whilst others may not be considered wants. For example, health promotion may be considered a need by health care workers but not perceived as such by many individuals.

It is unclear whether need is driving up the amount currently spent on medicines. Although a number of factors can be identified as contributing to the increased expenditure, few would appear to be needs-based:

- Changing patient demographics to a more elderly population
- Changing consultation rates and expectations
- Prescribing of expensive and/or inappropriate medicines
- Availability of drugs for new indications
- Increasing number of patients on long-term maintenance therapy

- More drugs initiated as a result of screening
- Development of new drugs that are more effective, safe and costly
- Increasing trend for multiple therapy
- Shift of care from secondary to primary care
- Successful marketing/promotional activity of the pharmaceutical industry
- Increased availability of social medicines

In response to the increased demand for medicines, a number of different approaches have been tried to reduce expenditure on medicines:

- Profitability of the pharmaceutical industry subjected to rigorous, on-going review;
- Public campaigns implemented to reduce demand for medicines by encouraging individuals to take greater responsibility for their own health, whilst making more medicines available for sale in pharmacies;
- Price sensitivity of prescribers improved by making them financially responsible for what they supply.

Given the inherent limitations of the above strategies and the ever-increasing demands for health care, rationing, or priority setting as it is sometimes euphemistically called, is inevitable. Rationing occurs at the national, local or individual level, and may involve one or more of seven possible strategies (4): rationing by denial, e.g. limited range of medicines available; rationing by selection; rationing by deterrence, e.g. prescription charge; rationing by deflection; rationing by delay, e.g. waiting lists; rationing by dilution, e.g. each patient gets less; and rationing by termination.

DETERMINING NEED

Historically, departments of public health have been empowered to determine and monitor the health needs of a given population. However, their assessment tools are relatively insensitive to need at the level of prescribing. There is limited available data (5) that suggests there are growing inequalities in prescribing, because need is not the main factor that influences the decision to use a medicine. Perceived need, particularly for a new medicine, is often fuelled by the pharmaceutical industry and the strength of their relationship with the prescriber, patient, patient self-help group and media. Whilst this situation may be unacceptable, the rationing process itself is not without concern. The responsibility for decision-making is becoming ever more diffuse, there is often little transparency in the decision-making process and there is a poor understanding of those who ration, e.g. secretary of state, local health groups/primary care groups or general medical practitioners.

Rationing the availability of medicines and postcode prescribing are not acceptable to many in the UK national health service. They may, however, remain unavoidable given the market structure of a health system that attempts to be free at the point of delivery. In essence the UK national health service, in common with other state run systems, has had to develop an alternative rationing system to that which operates in a free market based on the cost of the service or medicine. The inherent problem is that any alternative system must not reflect the fundamental inequalities in the income of individuals or other non-health-related characteristics. To be fair and equitable it must be needs-based, evidence-based and contain a society-based priority weighting. With such an assessment tool the medicines we need may well be affordable. The unresolved dilemma is to identify those who should differentiate need from want and be responsible for explicitly prioritizing need. Whatever the future strategy we must break with tradition and ignore decisions based on short-term financial issues and reject the philosophy that prescribing excellence equates with an underspend of allocated monies.

REFERENCES

1. Marinker M. *Controversies in Health Care Policies: Challenges to Practice*. BMJ Publishing Group: London, 1994.
2. Office of Health Economics. *Compendium of Health Statistics*. OHE: London, 1997.
3. Dixon J, Inglis S, Klein R. Is the English NHS underfunded? *Br Med J* 1999; **318**: 522–6.
4. Kleine R, Day P, Redmayne S. *Managing Scarcity: Priority Setting and Rationing in the National Health Service*. OUP: Buckingham, 1996.
5. Bradshaw N, Walker R. Equity of prescribing: a pharmaceutical issue. *Pharm J* 1997; **259**: R38.

8

Physician Choice or Patient Choice: Ethical Dilemmas in Science and Politics

ANDREW EDGAR

Centre for Applied Ethics, Philosophy Section, University of Wales,
Cardiff, UK

INTRODUCTION

The purpose of this chapter is to explore the balance that must exist between the physician and the patient in determining the patient's access to pharmaceuticals and other medical therapies. It is hardly novel to observe that the second half of the twentieth century has seen a fundamental challenge to the culture of medical paternalism, in which the physician—albeit in the supposed best interests of the patient—dictated the form of therapy which the patient would undergo. The recognition of a raft of patients' rights, the rise of patient advocacy groups, as well as increased patient involvement in determining the goals and values of medicine has fundamentally transformed medical culture. The decline of medical paternalism has, inevitably, served to make medical decision-making more complex, as the simple certainties of paternalism are replaced by increasingly problematic negotiations, and often negotiations between parties that share surprisingly little in the way of culture or knowledge. The complexity of the decision-making process reverts, at least in part, to the problem of determining what information and value positions can legitimately be brought to these negotiations. At its crux is the problem of determining when the position of one

Pharmaceutical Ethics. Edited by S. Salek and A. Edgar.
© 2002 John Wiley & Sons, Ltd.

or other of the parties has descended into irrationality, and is thus no longer defensible.

The chapter will proceed by rehearsing a defence of medical paternalism, and by critically exploring its justification in terms of both an underlying philosophy of medicine, and a political philosophy. It will be argued that an understanding of the process of negotiation that exists between physician and patient demands a fundamental reassessment of both the culture of medical science, and the political culture within which medical care is delivered. Only a position that recognizes the thoroughly cultural and value-laden nature of this negotiation can hope to untangle good and bad argument, and thus to reassess the balance of the contributions of physician and patient.

MEDICAL PATERNALISM AND THE LIBERAL STATE

Medicine exists, it may be assumed, to diagnose the medical needs of the patient, and to discover and apply appropriate therapies that will either remove the need, or at worst alleviate distressing symptoms. From this perspective, the question of whether medicine should be part of a state-controlled health care system, or should be left to the free market, is a question of the best way to realize this goal, rather than a question of whether or not profit-making can be the primary goal of medicine. A benign medical paternalism presupposes this goal of the alleviation of need, but it may be argued that it does so only by invoking, implicitly or explicitly, a particular understanding of the nature of medical science. It rests upon what is known as the biomedical model of medicine. Put briefly, this model interprets disease as a disruption in the normal functioning of the human organism. Normal functioning can be objectively determined, and with due awareness of differences in age, gender and the like, is universally applicable to the human species. The task of medicine is to restore the organism to its normal state. While this model has been much debated, not least in terms of the possibility of coherently determining the normal functioning of an organism in a given situation (1), if it can be coherently formulated, then it facilitates a definition of "medical need" in terms of that which will restore normal functioning. Medical paternalism can therefore rest upon the assumption that the physician has an expertise in diagnosing and treating the needs of the patient's body. There is no point in consulting the patient over the nature of the therapy, for the patient lacks expertise in diagnosis and treatment (so that, in consulting the physician, the patient hands over the care of their body just as they might hand over a damaged car or computer to a suitable technician). Perhaps more significantly, the patient does not have to be consulted over the goals of the treatment. If need is a divergence from normal functioning, and normality is an objective and universal condition of the human organism, then there is no space for negotiation over the goals of therapy. The patient cannot but want to be restored to the objectivity condition of normal functioning (just as the car or computer owner cannot but want their machine to function optimally).

This account of medical paternalism may be placed into a broader political context. It is generally assumed that a central task of the liberal state is to safeguard the rights—the freedoms—of its citizens. From the writings of John Locke (in the seventeenth century) onwards liberals have argued that citizens have rights to life and to health (2). Even a minimal interpretation of these rights would hold that the individual should be free from assaults, by other humans, that would endanger their bodily integrity. This may, first of all, be seen to provide the basis for the state's obligation to regulate the provision of medicine, whether that provision is through a national health system or a free market. Medicines are potentially dangerous products, and specialist expertise is required in order to administer them in therapeutic doses. The ordinary citizen lacks such expertise, and must therefore be protected, for example by the distinction between prescription and "over the counter" drugs, and by the requirement to research and document fully the maleficent and beneficent effects of pharmaceuticals.

Yet there are two deeper issues here. First, placing medical paternalism within a liberal context allows for a reinterpretation of the concept of "need". Liberalism is committed to giving the citizen the greatest possible scope to pursue their freely chosen goals and activities. The better the health of the individual, which is to say, the closer they are to normal functioning, then the greater opportunity they will have to pursue a wide range of goals. Disease inhibits one's freedom. The satisfaction of needs may thus be understood as the prerequisite to all other human activities, and indeed, to one's full participation as a citizen within the liberal state (3).

Second, Locke held the rights to life and health (and indeed other fundamental liberal freedoms) to be inalienable. That is to say that no one, including the citizen him or herself, could justly violate his or her own rights. The citizen is therefore not free to take their own life or to harm their own health. Such acts would be considered irrational, and the state has an obligation to protect the citizen from his or her irrational acts or decisions, just as it is obliged to protect citizens from the irrational acts of others. The patient's freedom of self-diagnosis may therefore be legitimately restricted to a few minor ailments and self-treatment restricted to medicines of relatively low toxicity. Conditions are made as hard as possible for the irrational citizen to harm him or herself with pharmaceuticals. Yet this restriction is ultimately determined by the medical profession. While it may regulate pharmaceutical production and the general provision of medicine, the state must also rely upon medical expertise to determine which pharmaceutical products are to be made available to the patient, and under what conditions. The liberal state therefore appears to reinforce, and indeed to be reliant upon, medical paternalism.

In summary, the above account of paternalism, from a biomedical and liberal perspective, serves to shift the balance between physician and patient—in any negotiation of the choice of a treatment—wholly to the physician, for any contribution from the patient is either superfluous (for the physician is expert in diagnosing and treating objective medical needs) or irrational (should the patient's opinion diverge from the physicians). Medical paternalism is benign, precisely insofar as it is protecting the patient from their own irrationality.

If the above account is plausible, then liberal philosophy supports paternalism. However, liberalism is historically also a source of the challenge to paternalism. Liberalism, in its defence of the primacy of individual freedom, stresses the autonomy of the rational individual. Such a rational being is capable of making free and informed decisions about his or her own life and the course it should take, and not least because the individual is deemed to be the best (and indeed only) judge of their own interests and preferences. This perspective may be used to ground the recognition of patients' rights and patient advocacy against paternalism. At its most minimal level, the limits to the expertise of the physician are exposed in the physician's lack of knowledge of the subjective experience of the patient's illness. While the physician may be an expert in the diagnosis and treatment of the disease in general, only the patient knows how they feel in suffering this particular bout of the disease now. Adequate diagnosis and treatment must, therefore, be conducted in open communication with the patient. More profoundly perhaps, a recognition of the uniqueness of the individual may also expose the fundamentally experimental nature of medicine and therapeutics (4). Each human is unique, both genetically and in terms of their life history. The fact that a treatment is effective on one group of humans does not mean that it will be effective (or even non-maleficent) to the next individual. The reporting of the subjective experience of therapy is therefore vital in respecting the patient's rights to life and health. Finally, the substantial literature on, and widespread practical implementation of, the idea of informed consent begins to recognize that the patient does have a role in medical decision-making (5).

While the liberal model begins to erode paternalism, it may be suggested that it does so from a weak foundation. This can be outlined from the example of informed consent. For all its importance in modern medical ethics, its defence is problematic. On the one hand, it allows increased recognition of some of the decisions with which the patient can be involved. Most notably, good information about the consequences and risks of treatment can allow the patient, quite rationally, to refuse certain forms of treatment—if, for example, they consider that the risk of side-effects, judged by them to be unpleasant, is not sufficiently outweighed by the probability of recovery. This in turn problematizes the idea of medical need. The patient may legitimately judge that they do not need certain treatments, so that need ceases to be simply a matter of objective expert judgement. More precisely, while both sides may recognize that the patient needs therapy, they do not have to agree that the patient needs this particular therapy. This disagreement can be rational, insofar as both have reasonable interpretations of available evidence on risk and side-effects. The patient judges that, for them, the risk is too great (perhaps because their behaviour is, in general, risk-averse, or they find the particular side-effects distressing). Again, the patient is being credited with the autonomy to be the best judge of their own interests, and thus their interpretation of risk overrides that of the physician.

On the other hand, informed consent still presupposes an issue of expertise. The patient must have some competence to understand the information presented to them. The sceptical critic of informed consent might then conclude that it is largely illusory. Truly informed consent would require the expert knowledge of the physician (so that even a physician would be unable to give informed consent to treatment outside of his or her own specialism). Disagreements between physician and patient could therefore still be resolved by decreeing the patient to be, if not irrational, then at least incapable of being informed or of understanding the relevant information. This is, in effect, to ask at which point the patient's interpretation of risk ceases to be reasonable. It is not clear how reasonableness can be assessed, if there is a dispute, other than by reverting to the expertise of the medical profession. As such, paternalism is reinstated.

SELF-INTERPRETING ANIMALS

The weakness with the liberal position, and crucially its weakness in allowing us to determine the rationality of the contributions of physicians and patients to negotiations, may lie in the picture it offers of how humans make and negotiate decisions. As has been implied above, in its defence of individual freedom, liberalism presupposes that humans are self-interested and typically rational beings, capable of identifying the goals that they, as individuals, wish to pursue and the most appropriate ways of pursuing them (6). It is generally wrong to prevent an individual from pursuing goals that have been chosen autonomously, or to assume that you know better than the individual what lies in their best interests. Typically the liberal argues that the freedoms of a citizen can only legitimately be curtailed when the exercise of those freedoms begins to infringe upon the freedom of others.

The liberal state thus strives to be neutral to the diverse choices of goals and interests that its citizens might make. But if the doctrine of the inalienability of rights is held, then certain goals (for example, committing suicide, or selling oneself into slavery) are not permissible, because in violating fundamental rights they cannot be the choices of rational beings. There is thus a limit to the neutrality of the liberal state.

It is of course possible to reject the doctrine of inalienability in order to restore neutrality, but that may only deepen or shift the problem. Inalienability allows an argument to be resolved by questioning the rationality of one or other of the parties involved. Prima facie, it is in the nature of argument that it should be resolved in favour of the superior rationality of one position. Without some device to assess rationality, all the parties involved are doing little, if anything, other than expressing subjective preferences. If a patient, for example, were to refuse treatment, there would be nothing more to say. It would be pointless to ask for reasons, for mere preference would be enough. Medical paternalism would be overcome, but only by reducing concern for one's health to little more than a matter of personal whim. The liberal aspiration to protect the individual from their own foolishness and ignorance does, intuitively, seem well grounded. The point then is not to reduce decision-making to the exercise of subjective preference, but rather to develop a model of decision-making that is richer and more appropriate to the medical context, so that it is clear exactly what might make for the foolishness and ignorance in a decision.

This model, it may be suggested, can be found in the work of the Canadian philosopher Charles Taylor (7). Taylor argues that human beings must be understood as cultural beings, who use complex languages to articulate their emotional lives, and thus to articulate their sense of what it is, morally, to be human. Humans are "self-interpreting animals". Consider the following: I am asked to choose tea or coffee. I choose coffee, and if asked to justify my choice, all I can do is report that I enjoy the taste of coffee more. There is nothing more to be said, and there is certainly no space for rational argument or negotiation. Another cannot rationally convince me that I really prefer tea. This is an example of what Taylor calls "weak evaluation". I act immediately upon my desires, and act so as to maximize my pleasure. However, if I am asked to choose between a fair trade brand of coffee (where profits are distributed back to the producers in the developing world) and another brand, matters of personal preference as to the taste of the coffees seem less pressing. Indeed, if I were to defend my choice of the non-fair trade coffee simply on the grounds that it tasted better, I might be suspected of a certain superficiality in my moral perspectives. For Taylor there are certain issues where weak evaluation is insufficient. A person cannot simply act upon their desires, but must rather find resources by which to evaluate those desires (in what Taylor calls "strong evaluation").

To analyse this distinction Taylor considers the emotional life of humans. The emotions that a person experiences at a particular moment will depend upon their understanding of their current situation, or perhaps a remembered situation. To be fearful, for example, presupposes that the person believes, rightly or wrongly, that there is an object (or event) to be feared out there. Fear is an emotion that is, presumably, not unique to humans. Animals may be afraid. To feel ashamed is slightly different. It will again rest upon a certain understanding of the situation in which the person finds themselves, but now that understanding is not simply of the existence of some external object or event. It is rather, a matter of self-understanding. To feel ashamed presupposes that the person recognizes or imagines that they have done something (or perhaps have some physical or emotional characteristic) that falls short of the ideal which they set for themselves, or which others expect of them.

The person who cheats in a game of soccer may come to feel ashamed, if they recognize that such behaviour falls short of an ideal of sportsmanship (or sportswomanship) to which they should aspire. An animal could not have this emotion, for it requires human language for its articulation and communication. I can explain and communicate my fear, fairly effectively, by dumbly pointing to the fearful object hurtling towards me. I cannot explain my shame simply by showing a video of my furtive handball. Only in a complex culture could that act be shameful, and indeed others may not share my interpretation. The reasonableness of my shame can be negotiated. Others may argue that my ideals are too lofty or too old-fashioned; that everyone acts that way; that in any case I should play to the whistle and if the referee missed the foul, then I am free to take advantage, and so on.

In effect, in committing the foul I acted immediately upon my desires. In feeling ashamed, I reassess those desires, as somehow unworthy of me. So, the person who chooses coffee purely on its taste is acting immediately upon their desires. The point is whether these desires are worthy. The choice can be negotiated, and a person who puts their own, fairly minimal, comforts over and above issues of justice may be condemned for being morally superficial.

Taylor's point is that there are certain emotions that only language-using beings could have, for example, pride, humility, indignation. Animals and humans can share the immediate desires that are the stuff of weak evaluation. Only humans have an emotional life that rests upon the evaluation of these desires (as to whether or not they are a worthy or unworthy basis of action). These emotions are, in Taylor's terminology, "subject-referring". That is to say, the emotion depends upon a conception of what the ideal (or good) life for a human subject may be. The articulation of this ideal requires language, both insofar as much of the ideal may be expressed to a significant degree in story telling and the use of examples, and in that such terms as "shame" can only be explained through a network of other concepts (e.g. cheat, liar, dishonourable, cowardly, undignified). Again, the point is that shame cannot be defined ostensibly. I cannot simply point to the shameful behaviour, because it is only shameful in terms of a specific understanding of the meanings and intentions of the actors involved. Others may perform exactly the same physical motions, and yet not experience shame. To describe a handball as furtive already calls upon the complex language that we use to ascribe motivations to ourselves and others. The emotion therefore depends upon resources one has to interpret the world, and crucially to interpret oneself.

FROM VOLUNTARY AMPUTATIONS TO ALTERNATIVE MEDICINES

Taylor is therefore offering a view of what it is to be human that is, to some degree, at odds with both the biomedical model and with liberalism. The biomedical model reduces humans to biological organisms (at least for the purposes of medical care). The liberal celebrates the rational autonomous individual as the best, and perhaps only judge of what is in their own best interests. Consider the following examples. Some people indulge in the activity of self-harming (for example deliberately cutting and scarring themselves, or by engaging in sadomasochistic activities). Others have presented themselves for surgery, requesting the amputation of healthy limbs, on the grounds that they are not able-bodied people and that the healthy limbs are a burden and cause of distress to them. The biomedical and liberal responses would seemingly concur in regarding such people as irrational. To impair, deliberately, one's normal biological functioning runs counter to the clear goals of medicine, and would seem to restrict one's freedom (if normal functioning is the precondition for all other human activity). Medical paternalism would therefore appear to be legitimate in protecting such people from themselves.

Taylor's account of the self-interpreting animal opens up a further perspective. For Taylor, the human being, even as a patient, cannot be reduced to a mere biological entity, for that biological existence is necessarily culturally interpreted. Normal functioning cannot merely be a matter of scientific fact. To use an obvious, if even slightly clichéd, example, one might here reflect upon the way in which epilepsy has been interpreted as both a disabling disease and as a divine gift in different cultures. More tellingly still, there has been much debate about the status of the deaf as a distinctive linguistic community (due to the presence of sign languages), so that the restoration of a deaf child to normal functioning (through cochlea implants) is seen as equivalent to the abduction of that child from his or her indigenous community.

Similarly, Taylor cannot share the liberal's conceit that an individual is the best judge of their own interests. The example of shame has already suggested that individuals are necessarily social creatures, using their awareness of how others judge them to judge themselves. Individuals do not passively submit to the judgements of others, but rather have the potential to negotiate those judgements. Such negotiation proceeds, implicitly or explicitly, by articulating ideals of what human life can be.

The self-harmers and voluntary amputees therefore pose a fundamental challenge to both the biomedical model and to liberalism. At the root of this challenge is a question of the relationship of the body to the good human life. The imposition of the medically ratified idea of normal functioning upon patients rules out self-harm and voluntary amputation as illegitimate (and thus irrational) lifestyles. It presupposes that the human ideal requires as healthy a body as possible. Self-harm and voluntary amputation ask whether an image of the good life can be articulated that includes, not merely the tolerance of a loss of physical integrity (as with genetic or accidental disability), but its active embrace. Such an image might be articulated in stories and especially in autobiographies, and the crucial question is whether or not such stories could make sense within—and indeed, could legitimately expand—our current interpretations of human life. The self-harmer and amputee are attempting to make us all understand the world differently.

The point here is not that the self-harmer and voluntary amputee will necessarily succeed in having their views of the good incorporated into our interpretations. Negotiation may result in the self-harmer and voluntary amputee still appearing to be irrational (and as such in need of psychiatric therapy). But if this is the result, then it cannot rest upon the mere dogmatic assertion of normal functioning, nor yet the dismissal of the self-harmer's and amputee's choices as mere whims. Rather, the issue is one of strong evaluation, and as such requires the discovery of some way of assessing the worth of the desires of the self-harmer and amputee. That assessment must allow the self-harmer and amputee scope to articulate their emotional lives—and hence the importance of storytelling and autobiography—but also allow an equally articulate response in terms of the richness, validity, perversity, superficiality or whatever of the self-harmer's and amputee's accounts. Such negotiation is perhaps never final. One cannot, for example, merely assert that the self-harmer is perverse, for that judgement itself needs defence and articulation (and ultimately rests upon what our language and culture allows us to say and feel about the human condition). What is important is that negotiation has proceeded through an enrichment of our understanding of the part that bodily health plays in the good life, and thus of what the good life might be.

Typically, it may be suggested, the liberal and biomedical models are not challenged. The physician and the patient are part of a common culture. The physician's ideas of normal functioning and the patient's are coterminous. Further, in many examples of medical care, the patient may be incapable of participating in decision-making, because of their medical condition. In acute or emergency care, issues of dignity and respect are largely beside the point. If patients can express emotion and desire, then they remain at the level of weak evaluation, concerned with pain or the fearful prospect of permanent injury or even death. It is thus, perhaps, to extreme cases that one must turn to explicate the potential conflict of physician and patient.

The much used example of a Jehovah's Witness refusing a life-saving blood transplant is highly relevant here, but consider the following: a 20-year-old woman has been brought up in a strong religious tradition, akin to that of the Jehovah's Witnesses, that as part of its rich and complex belief system prohibits certain medical interventions. Yet the woman is also in contact with modern Western culture and in most outward respects lives as a typical middle-class Westerner. She suffers a life-threatening injury or illness that can only be effectively treated by one of the prohibited treatments. Needless to say, she wants to go on living. From the biomedical and liberal perspective it may be suggested that the only rational option is for the woman to take the treatment. To refuse treatment entails that the physical preconditions for any form of lifestyle are removed. Taylor's perspective is more subtle. The woman's religious upbringing is not a mere lifestyle choice (akin to taking up a hobby, or using one supermarket chain rather than another). The woman's religion provides much of the language and imagery through which she articulates her emotional life and thus her understanding of exactly who and what she is. In her religion is found the ideal of the good human life, through which she can engage in strong evaluation. The person she is cannot exist independently of this religion. If she takes the treatment she may live as a biological organism, but she will die as an adherent of her religion. The person she currently is will be destroyed. The initial point to make, therefore, is that, contra liberalism and the biomedical model, mere biological functioning is not necessarily the precondition to all other choices. The desire to go on living can, against liberalism's defence of the inalienability of the right to life, be subject to strong evaluation, and found to be an unworthy motivation for action.

In the example, it was suggested that the woman, despite her religious upbringing and adherence, still largely adopts a Western lifestyle. This, quite deliberately, complicates the issue. The woman has a more complex choice for she has two cultures and two languages through which to articulate her sense of personal identity. It may be suggested that this is not unusual. People do not generally belong to simple, homogeneous communities, but rather move, physically and emotionally, between complementary and often competing communities. Much of the richness of our emotional lives (not least as it is articulated in the high and popular arts) comes from our ability to draw upon diverse cultures, experienced directly, or indirectly through the reports of others. In this example, illness exposes a crisis in personal identity. The woman has, in her familiarity with Western culture, a language which will, in strong evaluation, defend the desire to life. It is, in effect, the language of the biomedical model and liberalism (and hence, again, indicates that the typical values of physician and patient will be coterminous). The woman could therefore go on living as a Westerner, suppressing her religious upbringing, or more profoundly, finding a way to Westernize her religious belief, re-articulating, in the language of Western liberalism, the truths of her religion. This is no small demand, and no doubt beyond the ability or strength of most. The point to be made, though, is that illness and disease may be significant precisely in that they demand, on the part of the patient, a reinterpretation of who they are. The ambiguities and contradictions of a cultural inherence may be brutally exposed in the choices that have to be made. The choices cannot be avoided by a mere deferral to the dominance of the liberal or biomedical model. This is particularly the case in chronic illness, where, as Frank has shown, the illness cannot be treated as a mere hiatus in the routine course of one's life, with medical intervention serving to restore the patient to normal functioning, but rather something that has implications for one's self-understanding (for example, as chronically ill or in remission) (8).

A final example is perhaps of most relevance to the provision of pharmaceuticals. Alternative or complementary medicines are increasingly popular amongst patients. Many alternative treatments, such as homeopathy, are regarded as being of no therapeutic value by physicians. From the liberal biomedical perspective, and thus from the viewpoint of medical paternalism, the consumption of alternative medicines may be faintly puzzling—why take homeopathic cures when proven orthodox treatments are available?—but, providing there is no proven toxicity, permissible. The consumption of alternative medicines would be seen as being the result of an exercise of consumer preference, and if the consumer wishes to spend their own money (but not the state's) on these compounds, then they are, after all, the best judge of their own desires and how to satisfy them. There may be problems only if alternative medicines are taken instead of effective orthodox treatments, so that the patient's health suffers. At that point the choice comes to appear to be irrational, not least because the patient has ceased to make a properly informed choice about their own health care. Such an approach relies upon the biomedical model, precisely in that it assumes all that is important of a medicine is its proven efficacy in the treatment of a biological condition.

It may be suggested that the appeal of alternative medicines is more profound than a mere subjective whim on the part of the patient. Regardless of their efficacy, much alternative medicine is believed to be safer, more natural, and generally more comprehensible to the patient. The validity of these beliefs is, for the moment, beside the point. The use of alternative medicine expresses a deep distrust of orthodox medicine on the part of the patient. Precisely in its scientific and technological complexity, its seeming reduction of the patient to a mere biological entity, and thus its paternalism, orthodox medicine alienates the patient. This is, again, an issue of strong evaluation. Orthodox medicine violates some people's understanding of what it is to be human, stripping them of dignity and autonomy. To debate the merits of orthodox and alternative medicine simply in terms of their relative efficacy will, ultimately, be to talk at cross purposes, for that debate presupposes, on the part of the physician, the very matter that should be open to discussion: the nature and status of science (and particularly medical science) itself. Belief in the safety and naturalness of alternative therapies may be naive, but that naiveté needs to be articulated, and crucially the root desire of the advocates of alternative medicine—for treatments that are safe and comprehensible—may not readily be dismissed as irrational (even if it might presently be impractical).

CONCLUSION

Medical paternalism is not straightforwardly a bad thing. Physicians have a specialist scientific knowledge that often cannot readily be shared with patients. There are situations in which a physician's choices will, unproblematically, take precedence. For example, in emergency care, where the patient is incapable of expressing an opinion, or where the patient's expressed opinion is clearly distorted by mental illness or depression. In other, routine treatments, the patient simply may not wish to express an opinion or to challenge the physician's choice. The patient may routinely hand themselves over to the physician's care, confident that they share with the physician a common perception of the activities and goals of medicine. Similarly it has been acknowledged that the state does have an obligation to protect its citizens from their own irrationality and illness, and medical expertise may be vital in identifying such incompetence.

Yet it has been suggested that in its association with the biomedical model, medical paternalism is problematic for it tends to reduce the patient to a mere biological organism, stripping them of their humanity. Failing to respect another's humanity removes the ground from which any divergence between the physician's and the patient's

Continues

Continued

perception of what medical care is may be raised. The possibility of what Taylor has called "strong evaluation" is thus inhibited. The concept of "strong evaluation" suggests that disputes between physicians and patients crucially turn upon the understanding of what it is to be human, and not least upon the recognition of the part that health and bodily integrity play in that understanding.

It has been suggested that modern paternalistic medicine, like modern liberalism with which it has a certain coherence, presupposes an impoverished view of what it is to be human. Those who, for whatever reason, are out of step with such modernity, are likely to find their choices being traduced as irrational. Again, it must be stressed that not all positions are equally rational. Strong evaluation will expose the choices of some parties to be superficial, naive, arrogant or perverse. But such exposure will occur only if it is recognized that medicine is unavoidably part of human culture, and that the physician's choice cannot prevail by a dogmatic appeal to the apparent objectivity of scientific expertise.

REFERENCES

1. Boorse C. Health as a theoretical concept. *Philos Sci* 1977; **44**: 542–73.
2. Locke J. *Second Treatise of Government*. Kackett: Indianapolis, 1980 (originally published in 1690).
3. Daniels N. Health-care needs and distributive justice. *Philos Public Affairs* 1980; **10** (1): 147–76.
4. Badcott D. A Philosophical Study of Some Aspects of the Equivocal Nature of Therapeutics. Unpublished PhD thesis, University of Wales, Cardiff, 1999.
5. This volume, chapters 5 and 6.
6. Rawls J. *A Theory of Justice*. Oxford University Press: Oxford, 1972.
7. Taylor C. Self-interpreting animals. In *Human Agency and Language: Philosophical Papers I*, Taylor C (ed). Cambridge University Press: Cambridge, 1985.
8. Frank AW. *The Wounded Story Teller*. University of Chicago Press: Chicago, 1995.

9

The Economics of Drug-Related Morbidity and Mortality: Ethical Considerations

J. LYLE BOOTMAN AND AMY J. GRIZZLE

Center for Health Outcomes and PharmacoEconomic Research, University of Arizona, College of Pharmacy, Tucson, AZ, USA

INTRODUCTION

During the last decade, there have been many important changes within the health care systems around the world. Advancements in technology have been responsible for extending life, but have also resulted in escalating health care costs. Policy revisions throughout the world have also mandated changes in the way scarce resources are allocated and health care is delivered. An aging population has also contributed to the problem of rising health care costs. Most significant in the US is the "corporatization of health care". Simply stated, providers are increasingly employees for large for-profit health organizations. Even more striking is the fact that "Fortune 500" employers have become the major purchasers of health care.

In 1990, US health care costs (US$650 billion) represented 12% of the gross national product (GNP) (1). During the next decade, the proportion of health care spending had been steadily increasing, with 15% (US$998 billion) in 1994 and a projected health care expenditure of 20% (US$1.75 trillion) of GNP by the year 2000. Similar statistics and growth exist for most

Pharmaceutical Ethics. Edited by S. Salek and A. Edgar.

developing countries (1). The need for balance between health care costs and quality of care is an issue throughout the world.

It has become apparent that as a major consequence of this economic and environmental change there is an increasing need for pharmacists to better understand and better assess the literature with regard to the economic, as well as the clinical, aspects of drug therapy. Understanding the factors that drive health care costs is the first step in evaluating and solving this problem. Drug-related morbidity and mortality has recently been identified as a costly outcome of pharmaceutical treatment, contributing substantially to the rising health care expenditure. The purpose of this chapter is to discuss the extent to which drug-related problems (DRPs) can be quantified and valued, examine the ethical issues surrounding their occurrence, and explore possible solutions for prevention of drug-related morbidity and mortality.

Drugs are administered for the purpose of achieving definite outcomes, such as curing disease, reducing or eliminating symptoms, retarding or halting disease progression, or preventing illness or symptoms (2). Whenever drug treatment is given, there is the potential for sub-optimal outcomes that diminish a patient's quality of life. One such example is the occurrence of DRPs. A DRP is defined as an event or circumstance involving drug treatment that actually, or potentially, interferes with patients achieving an optimal therapeutic outcome (2). Hepler concluded that a major function of the pharmacist is to enhance and maintain the quality of drug therapy and, thus, reduce the risk of drug-related morbidity. Pharmacists must be committed to preventing and resolving DRPs. Drug-related problems can be classified into eight categories as follows (2):

1. **Untreated indications**. The patient has a medical problem that requires drug therapy (an indication for drug use) but is not receiving a drug for that indication.
2. **Improper drug selection**. The patient has a drug indication but is taking the wrong drug.
3. **Sub-therapeutic dosage**. The patient has a medical problem that is being treated with too little of the correct drug.
4. **Failure to receive drugs**. The patient has a medical problem in which a drug was prescribed but is the result of not receiving a drug (e.g., for pharmaceutical, psychological, sociological, or economic reasons).
5. **Overdosage**. The patient has a medical problem that is being treated with too much of the correct drug (toxicity).
6. **Adverse drug reactions**. The patient has a medical problem that is the result of an adverse drug reaction or adverse effect.
7. **Drug interactions**. The patient has a medical problem that is the result of drug–drug, drug–food, or drug–laboratory interaction.

8. **Drug use without indication**. The patient is taking a drug for no medically valid indication.   *Off Label usage*

Drugs are widely recognized as a valuable contribution to the prevention and resolution of disease. Unfortunately, the overall value of drugs diminishes as they transition from pre-marketing to post-marketing status. The occurrence of DRPs will always be greater once a drug is approved and administered in a "real world" setting, i.e., outside of randomized controlled clinical trials. This difference in the incidence of DRPs is responsible for the decrement in value. Strategies need to be employed to minimize this gap and ensure that the ultimate value of drugs is achieved.

QUANTIFYING THE PROBLEM: THE COST OF DRUG-RELATED PROBLEMS

Much of the literature to date describing DRPs and their economic consequences focused on hospitalization secondary to adverse drug effects or medication non-compliance (3). Sullivan et al. (4) surveyed available literature and, using a meta-analytic technique, estimated that non-compliance accounted for 5.3% of hospitalizations; direct medical costs associated with these hospitalizations were estimated to be US $8.5 billion. The authors estimate an additional US $17 to $25 billion in indirect costs related to drug therapy non-compliance. A more recent estimate puts the total costs of non-compliance at greater than US $100 billion (5).

Drug-related problems occurring during hospitalization are also common. Bates et al. (6,7) conducted a six-month prospective cohort study evaluating over 4100 hospital admissions. The authors reported a rate of 6.5 DRPs per 100 admissions, with 28% of the problems preventable. These adverse events extended the length of hospital stay by 2.2 days, and were associated with increased costs of US $2595 per DRP. The authors estimated annual costs attributable to DRPs at US $5.6 million for their institution, of which US $2.8 million was due to preventable events.

In a more recent evaluation (8), Classen et al. performed a matched case–control study with 1580 cases and nearly 21,000 controls. Although the rate of DRPs per 100 admissions was lower than that found by Bates et al. (2.43 versus 6.5), the increase in length of stay and costs per event were similar. Classen reported an increased length of stay of 1.91 days, with increased costs of US $2262. Extrapolating these figures to the US population, DPRs occurring in hospitalized patients would cost US $1.56 billion annually. Using the higher event rate (DPRs in 6.5% of admissions) from the Bates et al. study, US costs increase to US $4.2 billion a year. In addition to these morbidity costs, Classen et al. found that DRPs were associated with an almost two-fold increase in the risk of death (odds ratio 1.88 95% CI, 1.54–2.22; $p < 0.001$). It is clear from these studies that DRPs in hospitalized patients are associated with prolonged length of stay and increased economic burden.

Studies of emergency departments (EDs) have shown that between 2.9 and 3.9% of ED admissions are directly related to DRPs (9). Dennehy et al. estimated total annual costs of these DRP-related admissions at US$602,597.

Bootman et al. (10) evaluated the occurrence and cost of DRPs in nursing facilities. Decision analysis was used, with event probabilities and DRP management estimated by an expert panel of consultant pharmacists and physicians. The panel estimated that without consultant pharmacist services, approximately 42% of nursing facility residents would have an optimal therapeutic outcome (absence of DRPs). The authors estimated the cost of managing DRPs in this patient population at US $7.6 billion annually. Furthermore, deaths attributable to DRPs were estimated to occur in 3 to 4% of nursing facility patients.

The most comprehensive study to date, conducted by Bootman and Johnson (11,12), suggests that DRPs in the ambulatory setting cost society approximately US$76 billion annually. Using an expert panel, they developed a model of therapeutic outcomes resulting from drug therapy and estimated the magnitude of drug-related mortality and morbidity in the US (excluding hospital DRPs). The largest component of the total cost comprised drug-related hospitalizations (62% of total cost), followed by admissions to long-term care facilities. Based on model estimates, more than 28% of hospitalization admissions result from drug-related morbidity and mortality. Additionally, the panel members estimated that approximately 60% of patients taking prescription medication would have an optimal therapeutic outcome. Recently, the analysis was updated and the estimated cost in 2000 was US$177.4 billion(13). All of these estimates lead to the same conclusion; drug-related morbidity and mortality is a common and costly problem facing society.

MEASURING OUTCOMES OF CARE

Avoiding DRPs is the central goal in achieving optimal therapeutic outcomes in patients receiving drug therapy. Patient outcomes can be divided into three broad categories: clinical, humanistic, and economic. Clinical outcomes are the traditional measures of efficacy applied in the evaluation of pharmaceutical products and services, e.g., cancer cure rate, time to fracture healing, incidence of myocardial infarction, reduction in pain severity, etc. Humanistic outcomes relate to patient quality of life, preference, and satisfaction. Evaluation of humanistic outcomes attempts to quantify and value health concepts such as pain and suffering, and the impact of treatment on patients' daily activities, physical and mental health. Economic outcomes are those focusing on resource consumption associated with achieving a particular outcome. These resources may encompass items such as physician visits, medication, hospitalization, laboratory tests, medical procedures, transportation, time lost from work, etc.

The ideal situation is when a therapy intervention improves all three of the above-mentioned health outcomes (clinical, economic, and humanistic) (Table 9.1, Scenario 1). A major ethical issue surfaces when one or more of these outcomes does not improve, but rather worsens as a result of treatment (Table 9.1, Scenarios 2–6). For example, suppose a drug reduces the incidence of myocardial infarction, but negatively affects patient quality of life due to side-effects such as depression, erectile dysfunction, and insomnia. In the total view, this drug is less cost-effective than alternative treatments to prevent myocardial infarction (Table 9.1, Scenario 2). In other words, it provides a negative economic outcome. Although it achieves the targeted clinical outcome (prevention of myocardial infarctions), one must ask whether treatment with this medication is ethical. This is an example where the three outcomes (clinical, economic, humanistic) are not affected in the same direction, precipitating an ethical dilemma. Sacrificing patient well-being to achieve a clinical endpoint cannot be considered a successful therapeutic outcome. Health, after all, encompasses more than the physical dimension; patient satisfaction, mood, vitality, and attitude can have a substantive impact on response to treatment and overall health. As health care professionals become increasingly aware of the need to balance these desired outcomes, drug development and evaluation will focus on the patient as a whole, rather than partitioning these outcomes for assessing treatment. As we develop more valid and reliable tools to evaluate the three outcomes, these inconsistencies will be more apparent. The result will be an increase in the debate centered around ethics.

Furthermore, evaluation of clinical, humanistic, and economic outcomes raises the concern about balancing the cost of care with the quality of care. Access to health care must also be considered when determining the value of pharmaceutical products and services. These three entities (cost, quality, and access) are closely intertwined; changes in one area have a direct impact

Table 9.1   Examples of potential outcomes: scenarios resulting in ethical debate

	Clinical	Economic	Humanistic
Scenario 1	↑	↑	↑
Scenario 2	↑	↓	↓
Scenario 3	↑	↑	↓
Scenario 4	↑	↓	↑
Scenario 5	↓	↓	↑
Scenario 6	↓	↓	↓

on the other components of health care delivery. A recent Medicare report serves as an example, illustrating the relationship among these health care determinants (14). The Medicare report indicated that although routine preventive care is covered by the plan, few patients are receiving the services offered. Mammograms, for example, were provided for only 28.3% of women aged 65 to 69, despite recommendations for screening every other year in this age group. Regionally, mammogram rates in the US varied from 12 to 50%. Similarly, only 12% (rates ranged from 2.4 to 22.2% in the US) of Medicare recipients were screened for colorectal cancer, a procedure recommended annually for people over age 50. Researchers suspect that these statistics are linked to the wide variation in the quality of care from region to region and from doctor to doctor. Lack of a structured system, such as within health maintenance organizations, offers no way of assuring that the proper care is provided.

Variations in quality of care, in this case, have resulted in problems related to access of care. One could argue in the long run that this will result in increased health care costs. It seems obvious that shifts in quality and access would lead to changes in the cost to deliver care to this patient population and the ability to manage the consequences associated with their low adherence to preventive care.

In summary, understanding the relationships between cost and quality of medical interventions (i.e., drugs) from a total perspective is essential to making rational decisions as we develop better tools and information systems to measure the impact on outcomes (clinical, economic, humanistic). Ethical debate will become a prime focus of discussion relative to the allocation of resources and medical decisions.

APPROACHES FOR REDUCING DRPs

Given current estimates of the cost of DRPs, even small reductions in the occurrence of these adverse events would lead to considerable savings to the health care system. Policies and services should be developed to reduce and prevent drug-related morbidity and mortality. Several approaches for reducing DRPs will be discussed, including: 1. assessment of therapies via pharmacoeconomic analysis; 2. provision of pharmaceutical care; and 3. creating incentives for identifying and eliminating DRPs.

Pharmacoeconomic Analysis

Pharmacoeconomic evaluation is one methodology that can be employed to develop policies aimed at reducing DRPs and providing cost-effective patient care. Pharmacoeconomic research is becoming adopted as a health science discipline by the pharmaceutical industry, academic pharmaceutical scientists, and pharmacy practitioners throughout the world. It is generally defined as the description and analysis of the costs and consequences of pharmaceuticals and pharmaceutical services and their impact upon individuals, health care systems, and society (1). The research methods utilized by scientists in this emerging discipline are drawn from the economic and epidemiological disciplines.

Obviously, pharmacoeconomic research is but one of several new health areas of inquiry emerging as we approach the year 2000. It is proposed that this emerging discipline will have a dramatic influence on the delivery and financing of health care throughout the world. It is further suggested that pharmacoeconomics may influence health care and the practice of pharmacy at a magnitude equivalent to or greater than other relatively new disciplines such as clinical pharmacy and pharmacokinetics.

During the early 1960s, pharmacy began evolving as a clinical discipline within the health care system. It was during this time that pharmaceutical disciplines, such as pharmaceutics, clinical pharmacy, drug information, and pharmacokinetics, became a critical and integral part of pharmacy education and science. It was in the 1970s that the discipline of pharmacoeconomics developed its roots. The first article published in the pharmacy literature occurred in 1978. when McGhan et al. (15) introduced the concepts of cost–benefit and cost–effectiveness analyses. Interestingly, the actual term "pharmacoeconomics" was not put forth until a decade later (1987), when Townsend (16) described this evolving discipline (pharmacoeconomics) in pharmacy. To date much of the efforts in this discipline have been directed toward the refinement of the research methods and their application to evaluating pharmaceutical services and specific drug therapies.

Interestingly, during the past decade, "pharmacoeconomics" has become an important consideration in drug development and marketing by the pharmaceutical industry. Pharmacoeconomic studies attempt to identify, measure, and compare the costs (resources consumed) and consequences (outcomes) of pharmaceutical products and services (17). The research methods and tools such as cost-minimization, cost-effectiveness, cost–benefit, cost-of-illness, cost–utility, decision analysis, and quality of life assessment are included within this framework. In essence, pharmacoeconomic analysis employs tools for examining the impact of alternative drug therapies and services related to the drug treatment of patients (1).

In short, beyond the elements of a well-designed clinical trial, the additional component in a pharmacoeconomic evaluation is a system(s) to monitor or estimate: 1. medical care utilization or resource consumption (direct costs and benefits); 2. lost productivity through morbidity and/or premature death (indirect costs and benefits); and 3. impact of disease and treatment on quality of life (intangible costs and benefits).

It is suggested that pharmacoeconomics will obtain a high level of recognition when its application in the clinical setting is more complete. In other words, when pharmacy practitioners begin to apply the results of pharmacoeconomic research data to therapeutic decision-making, thus positively influencing patient outcomes, the discipline will become an increasingly critical component of the pharmacy curriculum. Likewise, it is further suggested that the successful implementation of "pharmaceutical care" will come about only with sufficient pharmacoeconomic research that adequately documents the degree to which the benefits of pharmaceutical care outweigh the costs associated with those services. In fact, the profession of pharmacy is unlikely to succeed in its role of providing pharmaceutical care without this critical body of knowledge. Pharmacists must become the key players in assuring that drug therapy and related pharmacy services are not only safe and effective, but cost-effective as well.

Because pharmacoeconomic research includes the appraisal of all costs and outcomes, the impact of DRPs is evaluated and balanced against the beneficial effects of treatment. This type of valuation is critical in determining acceptable levels of negative outcomes in patient care. Obviously, some untoward effects can be traded off for desirable ones. Pharmacoeconomic analysis is helpful in determining the point at which those trade-offs no longer outweigh the benefits. Keeping the focus on the patient is the only way to avoid unethical practice when making treatment decisions. Patient well-being and quality of life should always be included in the decision-making process.

It is important to include all aspects of DRPs when evaluating and selecting treatment options. In addition to the known side-effects attributable to drug therapy, an assessment of risks associated with extrinsic factors is essential. Patient non-compliance is of particular concern when estimating the incidence of DRPs. Overmedication may lead to drug toxicity, resulting in additional medical resource use and decrement in quality of life. Non-compliance (undermedication) may produce treatment failures, necessitating additional resource use in the absence of the desired outcome. All of the consequences associated with an intervention must be addressed in a pharmacoeconomic evaluation, and can assist pharmacists in identifying areas to target for prevention of DRPs. Pharmacists and other health care providers have the responsibility of anticipating potential deterrents to patients achieving optimal therapeutic outcomes. Patient counseling and follow-up should assist in appropriately managing therapy, and aid in avoiding preventable DRPs. Neglecting these patient care obligations will place patients at higher risk of experiencing DRPs.

Pharmaceutical Care

The profession of pharmacy continues to undergo change and re-evaluation of its mission. There is consensus that the mission of pharmacy practice should be defined as fulfilling the societal need for professionals to assure the safe and effective use of drugs. To meet this end, there is agreement that pharmacists need to assume greater responsibility for the management of drug therapy in order to ensure positive therapeutic outcome. In essence, the profession has adopted the provision of pharmaceutical care as the paradigm for the future practice of pharmacy (2,18).

Pharmaceutical care involves the process through which a pharmacist collaborates with a patient and other professionals (i.e., physicians) in designing, implementing, and monitoring a therapeutic plan that will produce specific therapeutic outcomes for the patient. This in turn involves three major functions: 1. identifying potential and actual drug-related problems; 2. resolving actual drug-related problems; and 3. preventing potential drug-related problems.

As previously discussed, the pharmacist has an obligation to implement the principles of pharmaceutical care to ensure appropriate drug use. It would be unethical to knowingly omit patient care information that could prevent or lessen the risk of DRPs. This falls under the realm of the ancient Hippocratic principle that in practising medicine no harm should be done to the patient. The real problem of DRPs is, after all, precisely the human one to which Hippocrates pointed. Assessing whether harm has been done will often be more effectively expressed in such terms as anguish, pain, misery, inconvenience, or patient quality of life (19). Disregarding these "softer" measures of treatment success can be considered an ethical issue to which health care providers must be accountable.

Combining Pharmacoeconomics and Pharmaceutical Care

In addition to applying pharmacoeconomic methods to evaluating drug therapies, it is equally important to use these methods to evaluate pharmaceutical care services. This will enable the profession to delineate which pharmaceutical care services are cost-effective in relation to each other so as to improve our efficiency in improving patient care. As an example, a very useful application of pharmacoeconomics is in determining the economic impact of pharmacists in reducing the extent and cost of DRPs.

Johnson and Bootman (20) conducted a study to assess the impact of pharmaceutical care on the incidence and cost of the estimated US $76 billion problem associated with drug-related morbidity and mortality. They estimated that pharmaceutical care would reduce the cost of DRPs by approximately US $45.6 billion. In addition, 119,656 deaths could be avoided. Providing pharmaceutical care would lead to an increase in the number of patients achieving optimal therapeutic outcomes due to drug therapy; from approximately 60% to nearly 84% of patients, an improvement in outcomes of more than 40%.

Harrison et al. (21) evaluated the cost-effectiveness of consultant pharmacists in managing DRPs at nursing facilities. By providing consultant pharmacy services, the panel estimated that the percentage of patients experiencing an optimal therapeutic outcome would increase from 42 to 60%. The average cost of obtaining an optimal therapeutic outcome was US $235 per patient without consultant pharmacy services, and US $162 with consultant pharmacy services. Incremental cost-effectiveness analysis demonstrated that for each additional optimal therapeutic outcome achieved with a consultant pharmacist, there was an average saving in the cost of DRPs of US $1034.

These are excellent examples of how the pharmacoeconomic discipline can assist in the justification of pharmaceutical care as a practice paradigm. Given these analyses, pharmaceutical care services may be viewed as very cost-effective in reducing the incidence and prevalence of DRPs.

Improved Reporting Systems

The goal of preventing DRPs raises additional ethical issues for specific practice settings. Hospitals and other institutions, for example, may face problems of under-reporting of drug-related morbidity and mortality (22). In addition to making patient safety a priority, many institutions operate under capitation or "fixed-fee reimbursement" systems, providing financial incentives to reduce drug-related morbidity and mortality. Developing reporting systems to identify and inform health care providers about the occurrence of DRPs is a crucial step in the process of managing and eliminating these unfavorable events.

SUMMARY AND CONCLUSION

Drug-related morbidity and mortality is a prevalent problem contributing to the rising cost of health care. Undetected by managers due to underdeveloped information systems, today they represent a major economic, clinical, and quality of life issue in health care. DRPs are estimated to cost the US more than US $177 billion yearly in the ambulatory setting alone, and most likely in excess of US $200 billion including the institutional setting. Strategies for reducing DRPs should be further refined and implemented. Pharmacoeconomic analysis is a useful tool for identifying and evaluating the costs and quality of life impact associated with DRPs. Employing pharmacoeconomic research, pharmaceutical care has been shown to have a substantial impact on reducing the occurrence of DRPs. It is estimated that over US $45 billion could be saved annually by establishing pharmaceutical care programs. Additionally, policies are needed that create incentives for developing accurate DRP reporting systems so that steps may be taken to improve overall patient care. Drug-related morbidity and mortality offers a unique opportunity to develop effective reporting and management systems, reduce health care costs, and improve patient care, safety, quality of life, and overall well-being.

REFERENCES

1. Bootman JL, Townsend RJ, McGhan WF. *Principles of Pharmacoeconomics*, 2nd edn. Harvey Whitney Books: Cincinnati, OH, 1996.
2. Hepler CD, Strand LM. Opportunities and responsibilities in pharmaceutical care. *Am J Hosp Pharm* 1990; **47**: 533–43.
3. Einerson TR. Drug-related hospital admissions. *Ann Pharm* 1993; **27**: 832–40.
4. Sullivan SD, Kreling DH, Hazlet TK. Noncompliance with medication regimens and subsequent hospitalization: a literature analysis and cost of hospitalization estimate. *J Res Pharm Econ* 1990; **2**: 19–33.
5. Task Force for Compliance. Noncompliance with medications: an economic tragedy with important implications for health care reform. Baltimore, MD, November, 1993.
6. Bates DW, Cullen DJ, Laird N et al. Incidence of adverse drug events and potential adverse drug events. *JAMA* 1995; **274**: 29–34.
7. Bates DW, Spell N, Cullen DJ et al. The costs of adverse drug events in hospitalized patients. *JAMA* 1997; **277**: 307–11.
8. Classen DC, Pestontnik SL, Evans RS, Lloyd JF et al. Adverse drug events in hospital patients. *JAMA* 1997; **277**: 301–6.
9. Dennehy CE, Kishi DT, Louie C. Drug-related illness in emergency department patients. *Am J Health-Syst Pharm* 1996; **53**: 1422–6.
10. Bootman JL, Harrison DL, Cox ER. The health care cost of drug-related morbidity and mortality in nursing facilities. *Arch Intern Med* 1997; **157**: 2089–96.
11. Bootman JL, Johnson J. Drug-related mortality and morbidity: an economic analysis. Final report submitted to the Coalition for Consumer Access to Pharmaceutical Care, Washington, DC, July, 1994.
12. Johnson JA, Bootman JL. Drug-related morbidity and mortality. *Arch Intern Med* 1995; **155**: 1949–56.
13. Ernst FR, Grizzle AJ. Drug-related morbidity and Mortality: Updating the cost - of-illness model. J Am Pharm Assoc 2001; 41:192–199.
14. Medicare blasted for inequity, inefficiency. *USA Today*, April 20, 1999.

15. McGhan WF, Rowland CR, Bootman JL. Cost–benefit and cost-effectiveness: methodologies for evaluating innovative pharmaceutical service. *AJHP* 1978; **35** (2): 133–40.
16. Townsend R. Post-marketing drug research and development. *Ann Pharm* 1987; **21**: 134.
17. Bootman JL, Townsend RJ, McGhan WF. *Principles of Pharmacoeconomics.* Harvey Whitney Books: Cincinnati, OH, 1991.
18. Commission to Implement Change in Pharmaceutical Education: Entry Level Education in Pharmacy: A Commitment to Change. American Association of Colleges of Pharmacy, Alexandria, VA, 1992.
19. Dukes GMN. Economic costs of adverse drug reactions. *PharmacoEcon* 1992; **1**: 153–4.
20. Johnson JA, Bootman JL. Drug-related morbidity and mortality and the economic impact of pharmaceutical care. *Am J Health-Syst Pharm* 1997; **54**: 554–8.
21. Harrison DL, Bootman JL, Cox ER. Cost-effectiveness of consultant pharmacists in managing drug-related morbidity and mortality at nursing facilities. *Am J Health-Syst Pharm* 1998; **55**: 1588–94.
22. Wagner JT, Meier C, Higdon T. A perspective from clinical and business ethics on adverse events in hospitalized patients. *J Florida MA* 1997; **84**: 502–5.

10

Holistic Approach in Choice of Pharmaceutical Agents: Ethical Responsibilities

SAM SALEK

Welsh School of Pharmacy Centre for Socioeconomic Research,
University of Wales, Cardiff, UK

Significant changes are taking place within society. For healthcare systems to remain effective in addressing the current needs of their clients, consideration must be given to newly evolving individual priorities. Changes in our communities, economies, ideas, relationships and personal perceptions of health are shifting values and expectations; these new outlooks must be reflected in healthcare decision-making as part of our professional ethical responsibility. Increasingly, patients are seeking greater autonomy and an improved quality of life as well as quantity of life. As a reflection of the move by healthcare professionals to accommodate these changing needs, the concept of a holistic approach to treatment decision-making must become an integral part of day-to-day healthcare delivery. Moreover, in an effort towards fulfilling our ethical responsibilities, there should be a complete shift from the more traditional approaches in medicine towards full patient orientation. It therefore becomes paramount to recognize the importance of evaluating the holistic approach to the treatment of patients, through attaching equal weight to clinical, humanistic and economic outcomes in the clinical decision-making process, including choice of pharmaceutical agents. In this chapter, basic principles and fundamental elements of the holistic approach to treatment decision-making, such as patient perspective, patient autonomy, patient choice, patient empowerment, paternalism and informed/active par-

Pharmaceutical Ethics. Edited by S. Salek and A. Edgar.
© 2002 John Wiley & Sons, Ltd.

ticipation, will be discussed in the hope of establishing a better understanding of our ethical responsibilities in such a process.

WHAT IS MEANT BY "HOLISTIC APPROACH" IN THE CONTEXT OF HEALTHCARE DELIVERY?

In essence the concept of the "holistic approach" in medicine could be encapsulated as looking upon the patient as a "person" not a "disease" and consequently any effort towards treatment should be focused on the individual not on the illness. Logically, it would be unthinkable to assume that any medical practitioner could initiate a treatment including choice of pharmaceutical product, without considering the patient as a whole person and someone who ultimately will have to submit to the consequences of the practitioner's decisions. Such a phenomenon places an uncompromising ethical responsibility on the part of the practitioner to adopt a systematic approach to establish an insight into the whole person. This is commonly achieved by placing emphasis not only on physical but also on mental, emotional and social functioning of the patient. It is understood, however, that in some situations this can be achieved by involving a multidisciplinary team in our holistic approach. In recent years such an approach has gained an unprecedented impetus in the delivery of healthcare in most developed and developing countries. Undoubtedly, there are lessons to be learnt from complementary medicine, where its practice and success is largely focused on the holistic approach. Absence of the holistic approach in conventional medicine involving both medical and pharmacy practitioners has resulted in numerous failures of treatments with pharmaceutical products. This will be further examined in later sections of this chapter.

WHOSE PERSPECTIVE? THE CONCEPT OF NORMATIVE STANDARD

Differences in perspective between the patient, relatives and healthcare professionals, in particular medical practitioners, on health and impact of disease and its treatment have been demonstrated by many published studies. For example, Jachuck et al. (1), in their study on the effect of hypertensive drugs on the quality of life, summarized the rating of quality of life as follows:

- All medical practitioners (doctors) reported that patients' quality of life had improved.

- Three-quarters (314) of relatives reported that patients' quality of life was worse.
- Patients: 48% felt better, 8% felt worse, 44% felt the same.

The question here is whose was the correct perception? The answer must surely be: those on the receiving end. These findings confirm the view that patients are often found to have a very different perception and understanding of treatment than that expected by healthcare professionals.

The role of patients as experts in non-medical aspects of their disease and the medical practitioners as experts in medical aspects of the disease must be distinctly recognized. Thus, treatment decision-making should be based on involving both, which will in turn yield optimized outcomes. Healthcare professionals must be urged, through the adoption of the holistic approach, to learn and understand the patient's perspective and promote multidisciplinary teamwork, putting the patient in the centre in an attempt to fulfil their ethical responsibility.

Understanding the concept of "normative standard" would help us to appreciate the importance of the patient's perspective in the process of treatment decision-making. Philosophically, the criterion "normative standard" is the one held by the individual and only he/she can provide an assessment of his/her own well-being. However, if an observer, e.g. healthcare professional, assesses the well-being of a patient, the result will be based on the observer's *normative standard* and not the normative standard of the individual. Similarly, any other surrogate assessment suffers from the same deficiency. Therefore, only the patient can provide a meaningful response, since the patient will be comparing the present perceived state of health with his own present perceived normative standard (2).

The importance of patient perspective in the process of care was recognized by Hypocrites 2000 years ago when he wrote: "In the art of medicine there are three factors, the disease, the patient and the doctor. The doctor is the servant of the art. The patient must co-operate in fighting the disease".

WHOSE DECISION? THE CONCEPT OF AUTONOMY AND QUESTION OF CHOICE

Healthcare systems have denied patients their autonomy for many decades. In recent years, however, patients have increasingly become interested in playing an active part in the treatment decision-making process for their condition. Naturally, this has led to patients reclaiming their autonomy in order to facilitate their desire to exercise their competency and active participation.

Of course, the birth of such a phenomenon is largely owing to the advancement in information technology that has brought about the era of consumer enlightenment. This has led to a gradual change of culture among healthcare professionals with respect to their historical practice of making unilateral treatment decisions without patient involvement. Increasingly, government and private organizations are bombarding patients with information about their condition either through personal contacts, different media or the environment of secondary/primary care using different techniques.

There now seems to be a political will and consensus on the need for more consumer information. In the UK, the Labour Party policy document "A Fresh Start for Health" supports the development of patient autonomy. This means a patient population that is more self-confident, more assertive and more knowledgeable. Furthermore, this document promotes the rights of patients to gain more information about choices of treatment and proposes that patients who are better informed about alternative forms of treatment and who participate in the management of their case are more likely to co-operate in beneficial changes and may contribute to a better prospect for a successful outcome. Access to the right information at the right time is a crucial ingredient of modern healthcare. Across the world there is growing interest in information about health and health services, and to keep the momentum, it is important to develop a culture among healthcare workers that promotes a positive attitude to patients' rights to give and receive information (3). These issues will be examined further in later sections of this chapter.

EMPOWERMENT OF PATIENTS

The empowerment philosophy is based on the premise that human beings have the capacity to make choices and to be responsible for the consequences of their choices. Empowerment is defined as "an educational process designed to help patients develop the right level of attitudes, skills, knowledge (ASK) and degree of self-awareness necessary to effectively assume responsibility for their health-related decisions".

Chronic disease care requires an educational approach substantially different from the traditional compliance-related approach (4). Self-management for diseases such as diabetes requires balancing many metabolic and lifestyle factors. Routinely, individuals with chronic diseases make many choices that affect their health for better or for worse (5). Being empowered thus means that patients have learned enough about their disease and the consequences of an effective management or the lack of it to enable them to judge the cost–benefit of adopting a wide variety of healthcare recommendations (4).

It would be hugely wrong to assume that medical practitioners letting go of some of their power, empowering patients and encouraging them to be partners would be more time-consuming. Conversely, it should lead to much faster shared understanding, greater patient satisfaction and improved health outcomes, as has been shown in the case of diabetes (6,7). However, it must be borne in mind and clearly understood that for patient empowerment to achieve the desired outcomes: 1. it must be born out of a systematic and sound process and 2. it must be developed and subsequently evolved as a way of thinking. Such processes must include provision of the appropriate information, training/education and take into account a change of culture in health systems influencing both healthcare professionals and consumers. These issues will be dealt with briefly below.

Information, Education and Training

Providing information to patients is a necessary condition for achieving the treatment aims for health and quality of life improvement (8). Also, information, if appropriate in format and delivery, could facilitate choice of treatment. Most governments hope that by encouraging individuals to take responsibility for their own health, they will empower patients to participate in decisions made about the management of their condition. There is no doubt that patients and their carers want and need more information about their health, their condition, treatment and outcomes, as well as information to support them in day-to-day living with long-term diseases (3,9–12).

There is variation among patients with regard to the amount and timing of information they desire. Although some may prefer to leave decisions to the health professionals, there is increasing evidence to suggest not only that patients want more information than they can get (9,13,14), but also that medical practitioners may overestimate the amount of information that they provide (13,14). Waitzkin (14) found that medical practitioners overestimated the time spent giving information by about a factor of nine. He also found that the characteristics of the patient influenced the amount of information presented to them, e.g. sex and social class. A communication gap extends from what patients want to know about their medicines to what they actually learn from their physicians and pharmacists—the patient heard me, but did he understand me? This failure of professional and ethical responsibility has serious implications for public health.

The uncertainties of patients who, for example, in the USA receive approximately 1.5 billion prescriptions a year contribute to the failure of many of them to benefit fully from their medications (11). Information about drug treatment is likely to influence compliance and therefore the efficacy of treatment: thus it is essential that patients have access to appropriate sources of accurate information (9). Let's look at some examples to illustrate the extent of the problem and reinforce the need for adopting a holistic approach.

For example, in the case of diabetes, usually 50% of patients are diagnosed, of whom 50% are compliant and consequently 25% of patients are effectively treated. In the case of asthma, less than 10% of patients use their medication technically as they should. In the case of hypertension, the compliance with medication is between 20 and 30%. Let's take this one step further: if we have a 95% chance of a patient being correctly diagnosed and a 95% chance of the patient receiving the right medication, but only a compliance rate of 50%, then shockingly, the maximum potential effect of the medication would be $95\% \times 95\% \times 50\% = 45\%$. SOMETHING HAS TO BE DONE. To put this into perspective, in a climate of ever-increasing demand on our healthcare resources, what a waste of resources, time and energy not to mention the burden of all those complications arising from non-treated chronic diseases. The situation here is no different to where a customer in a butcher shop pays for a kilo of meat but is actually given only 0.45 kilo. This analogy holds true but with the fundamental difference that underselling of meat by the butcher does not cause any harm and untoward effect on the customer. Whereas, compromising the maximum potential effect of medication by 55% may cause the patient incalculable harm. Thus, as part of our professional and moral responsibility, we must ask ourselves "for how long can we go on spending scarce resources on reimbursing expensive, new innovative pharmaceuticals without providing patients with any guarantee of getting the maximum effect of their respective treatment?" This could also wholly or partly be remedied by pharmacy practitioners adopting a holistic approach in their practice through the provision of pharmaceutical care (i.e. responsible provision of drug therapy for the purpose of achieving definite outcomes that improve the patient's quality of life) and pharmacist-led medicine management clinics.

Change of Culture

Recent development in empowering patients in an effort to give them a voice and enable them to register their preferences when they are given the opportunity to choose from a number of alternative treatments has inherently brought about a change of culture. What this means is that patients as well as health professionals are experiencing something they have never done before. However, in some situations, one wonders whether patients and health professionals are ready to take on this two-way responsibility. For a patient who had never been given the opportunity to express his/her opinion about his treatments, suddenly he/she has been asked to make a difficult choice. Similarly, for professionals who, by and large, believed in paternalistic decision-making for centuries, this process places enormous pressure and naturally demands a change of culture. It has been reported that when patients have been given the choices, they have turned to the doctor and put the onus on him by responding "whatever you think doc"!

Simply, the answer is that both patients and health professionals must be appropriately trained and educated and prepared for such a change of culture. Frankly, it would be totally unfair to expect them to perform in the way described above and for patients to take on decision-making responsibilities without facilitating such a process. We first must teach them how to walk before we can expect them to run!

PATERNALISM OR INFORMED PARTICIPATION

By and large there is as yet little practical application of policies to the realization of patient empowerment within the health services, and thus to the development of a "partnership culture" (i.e. equal informed participation of patient and medical practitioners in the process of clinical decision-making). While it is assumed that such a partnership culture in healthcare is desirable, it is important to recognize that such a culture can only develop with the commitment of the general public, patients and medical professionals. Thus attempts should be made to establish the scope of any such partnership that is generally acceptable, as well as identifying the barriers (e.g. information, attitudes and socioeconomic factors) that could potentially inhibit involvement, commitment and possible methods of overcoming them (such as the improved quality and relevance of information given and improved methods by which it is communicated). In order to identify the socioeconomic barriers to a partnership culture that may exist, the diversity of economic, social and cultural conditions in different regions must be examined. This approach will allow exploration of the differences in attitudes, informational requirements and degree of commitment to partnership in different urban and rural conditions. Particular attention must be paid to the differences between populations in areas of high urban employment and areas of urban decline (e.g. long-term unemployment). The opinions and beliefs of an individual are formed within a social and economic environment and are subject to revision and change in the light of one's own experience and contact with the experience of others.

The development of a condition over time raises questions about the information that a person diagnosed with the condition requires in order to take any form of responsibility for their care, including involvement in treatment decision-making. Thus, a partnership culture presupposes that communication is a two-way process, and that both sides to the communication (i.e. patients, lay carers and public on the one hand, and healthcare professionals on the other) must not only be able to provide information, but also be able to listen and receive information, acting upon it appropriately. Crucially, in challenging a traditional view of medical paternalism, it does not presuppose that the responsibility for decision-making must then fall disproportionately onto the patient. Within a partnership culture, both sides must be prepared to have their opinions and values challenged and either be able to correct those opinions and values, or provide a reasoned reply according to their expertise and experience.

A strategy should be developed in order to facilitate an initial dialogue between those involved in a partnership culture, serving to explore the most appropriate ways in which informed participation can be established. Particular attention should be paid to the potential role that each group would have in a partnership culture, for example, in the education and support of patients and the general public. (For example, the role of pharmacists as a potentially effective and efficient resource in public healthcare education, provider of pharmaceutical care and therapeutic outcomes monitoring is in need of further research and promotion.) Such a strategy would also serve to identify the barriers that professionals face to involvement in a partnership culture, whether these barriers are generated within a professional culture (for example, through a traditional commitment to paternalism and a professional resistance to greater patient autonomy), or through technical and practical difficulties, including a lack of training in or knowledge of appropriate communication skills. It may, however, be suggested that it falls to the medical practitioners to initiate and lead the process of change towards a partnership culture and seek to draw on their professional expertise in the handling of change, and in particular to facilitate the exchange of experience, ideas and techniques for communication between different healthcare professionals.

Such an initiative on the part of health professionals should be coupled with taking appropriate steps in motivating the patients to be proactive players in the process. Often, poor motivation is expressed through poor compliance with medication use and change in lifestyle requirements. Older patients, in particular those in residential homes, often show resistance to motivation (15). Intrinsically, there are certain factors such as low self-esteem and economic disadvantage that may contribute to being a poor motivator. There are, of course, those patients whose conditions are often socially unacceptable and lead to social stigmatization and labelling, which in turn increases their sense of poor self-esteem and low perceived sense of self-worth. Miller and Rollnick (16) state "... it is no longer sensible for a therapist to blame a client for being unmotivated to change, any more than a salesperson would blame a potential customer for being unmotivated to buy. Motivation is an inherent and central part of the professional's task".

However, the process should be seen as a collaborative activity and the patient should demonstrate at least some willingness to engage. I therefore submit that motivation should be seen as both the patient's and professional's responsibility, with a caveat that the professional can greatly or marginally influence the patient's motivation depending on the patient's past and present experiences. Prochaska and DiClemente (17) developed a model of how people change either by themselves or with the help of professionals (Figure 10.1). This process is seen as a circular continuum and it is assumed that people should not be perceived as an on or off switch, as absent or present, but as a continuous process.

Active Participation and Shared Decision-Making

The current climate in healthcare systems coupled with unprecedented maturity on the patients' part demands a move away from the traditional passive involvement of patients towards promotion of a patient's active participation in decision-making. Medical practitioners should adopt this approach and encourage active participation of their patients in treatment decisions (18). Of course, medical practitioners who engage their practice in such a manner should be rewarded for their time and the use of extra resources.

The consumerism movement of the 1980s encouraged people to make demands from public services including the NHS, but failed to emphasize reciprocal responsibilities. Thus, searching for ways in which such demand for healthcare can be managed (19) has led to a new movement which

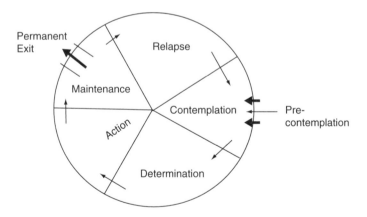

Figure 10.1 Model of how people change
Source: Adapted from (16).

emphasizes "shared decision-making" and "shared responsibilities". Shared decision-making has been viewed by the President's Commission for the Study of Ethical Problems in Medicine and Biomedical and Behavioural Research (20) as: providing relevant information about the clinical situation, alternatives, benefits and risks; assessing the patient's understanding; and giving the patient a clear opportunity to voice a preference. There are, of course, others who share the same sentiment (21–24).

Evidently a government's agenda is somewhat different from that of professionals and patients. They encourage self-help and informed choice

---

CASE STUDY

A few days ago I received a phone call from a 20-year-old female patient originally from Cardiff but currently a final year student reading radiotherapy in one of the medical schools in London and engaged in her clinical rotation in one of the oncology teaching hospitals. She has been suffering from pain (often excruciating) around her pelvic and abdominal area and so far clinical and differential examinations have been inconclusive. She is referred for a scan and waiting to hear. Her condition has interfered with her university and clinical rotation commitments. In the last visit to her general practitioner (GP) she was prescribed Prothiaden (dothiepin), a tricyclic antidepressant, and was told by her GP "I will give you a few tablets to ease your pain until you go for your scan". (This was all the dialogue that was exchanged between the medical practitioner and the patient.) On her way back to the hospital she stopped at a local pharmacy and obtained her medication. Later in the afternoon she looked-up the British National Formulary (BNF) in order to find out about the medicine she was prescribed. She was frightened by the fact that she was prescribed an antidepressant. She later went to the library in the hospital and found that a few scientific journal articles did not encourage the use of tricyclic antidepressants, in particular dothiepin, and also outlined its effect on cardiovascular systems, in particular as a risk factor for ischaemic heart disease. She immediately stopped taking the medication and was left angry because of the fact that her GP had not discussed with her that she was going to be prescribed antidepressants and why. She was given the impression by her GP that she was given a prescription for a painkiller. The end result was that the patient was left anxious, frustrated and totally lost faith in medical practice, not forgetting that her pain remained unresolved.

in the hope that it will translate into cost savings and a reduction in waiting lists (25). However, the time has come for a concerted action on everyone's part to form a partnership alliance in an environment of transparency and trust and start to treat the patients as "adults". For example, decisions for choice of pharmaceuticals, such as potentially toxic medications or initiating a diagnostic test that might require expensive or invasive techniques, must involve active participation of the patient. Active participation and a shared decision-making process is the product of a fully transparent and evidence-based dialogue between medical practitioner and patient, leading to a rational decision with high confidence of yielding optimized therapeutic outcomes (18). Undoubtedly, the absence of such a process would yield exactly the opposite, that is non-compliance, total resignation and loss of trust in health professionals. Perhaps a careful examination of one of my recent encounters with a frustrated patient would illustrate the validity of such a claim.

One school of thought argues that because little is known about the readiness of patients for active participation, shared decision-making may not work. Some claim that patients are not ready to take on responsibility and may not want to have an active role demanded from them. However, evidence exists that many patients wish to exercise their treatment preferences (26). Younger patients tend to be more critical of the paternalism approach in medical practice and more willing to have active participation in decision-making (26). But some older patients and some with serious conditions prefer to leave decision-making to the medical practitioner, perhaps because it allows them to avoid responsibility for the consequences of a wrong decision (27). However, a recent survey we carried out among 100 randomly selected patients with cancer from out-patients, in-patients and day care units (26 male, 74 female; median age 59 years, range 28–80) yielded somewhat different results. 71% of patients expressed a willingness to be involved in decision-making (Figure 10.2). Females were more likely to expect active involvement and those with breast cancer showed the greatest desire to play a role in decision-making. The age and education level of the patients did not influence their preferences.

This group of patients also expressed a greater need for information ($p = 0.009$). Furthermore, those patients who preferred to participate in decision-making experienced greater mental distress than those who preferred to leave the decision-making entirely to their doctors ($p = 0.04$). In contrast, patients expressed less mental distress when they felt highly informed ($p = 0.01$), reassured ($p = 0.001$), involved in the treatment decision-making process ($p = 0.006$) and their treatment was explained well ($p = 0.001$). In agreement with the previous body of evidence, these findings underpin the importance of patient active participation and shared decision-making and the urgency with which it must be implemented. We could

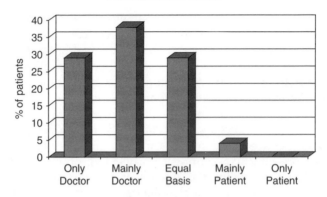

Figure 10.2 Patients' views regarding their willingness and level of involvement in treatment decision-making

go on and argue about the timing of such implementation but we must realize that "it always is too early, but suddenly it is too late".

CONCLUSION

A holistic approach in treatment decision-making in the context discussed in this chapter is the only way forward and also the only way that would ensure the fulfilment of our professional and ethical responsibilities.

REFERENCES

1. Jachuck SJ, Brierly H, Jachuck S, Wilcox PM. The effect of hypotensive drugs on the quality of life. *J R Coll Gen Pract* 1982; **32** (235): 103–5.
2. Osaba D. Measuring quality of life. *Progr Clin Biol Res* 1990; **354B**: 233–40.
3. Burns JP. Performance improvement with patient service partners. *J Nurs Admin* 1998; **28** (1): 31–7.
4. Feste C, Anderson RM. Empowerment: from philosophy to practice. *Patient Educ Counsel* 1995; **26** (1–3): 139–44.
5. Makoul G, Arntson P, Schofield T. Health promotion in primary care: physician–patient communication and decision making about prescription medications. *Soc Sci Med* 1995; **41** (9): 1241–54.
6. Greenfield S, Kaplan SH, Ware JE Jr, Yano EM, Frank HJ. Patients' participation in medical care: effects on blood sugar control and quality of life in diabetes. *J Gen Intern Med* 1988; **3** (5): 448–57.

7. Slowie DF. Doctors should help patients to communicate better with them. Letter. *BMJ* 1999; **319** (7212): 784.
8. NHS Wales. Better Information–Better Health. Government green paper, 1998.
9. Sims S, Golightly PW. Partnership with patients. Telephone helpline services can meet patients' demand for information. Letter. *BMJ* 1998; **317** (7155): 414.
10. Blenkinsopp A, Bashford J, Dickinson D. Partnership with patients. Health professionals need to identify how much information patients want. Letter. *BMJ* 1998; **317** (7155): 413–4.
11. Kessler DA. Communicating with patients about their medications. *N Engl J Med* 1991; **325** (23): 1650–2.
12. Ley DC. Caring for persons with AIDS: initiatives. The Casey House model. *J Palliat Care* 1988; **4** (4): 111–5.
13. Makoul GG. Perpetuating Passivity: A Study of Physician–Patient Communication and Decision Making. Unpublished Doctoral Dissertation, Northwestern University, 1992.
14. Waitzkin H. Doctor–patient communication. Clinical implications of social scientific research. *JAMA* 1984; **252** (17): 2441–6.
15. Furchtgott E, Wilkes Furchtogg M. *Aging and Human Motivation*. Plenum Series in Adult Development and Aging. Plenum: New York, 1999.
16. Miller WR, Rollnick S. *Motivational Interviewing*. Guilford Press: New York, 1991.
17. Prochaska JO, DiClemente CC. Transtheoretical therapy: toward a more integrative model of change. *Psychother: Theory, Res Pract* 1982; **19**: 276–88.
18. Braddock CH 3rd, Fihn SD, Levinson W, Jonsen AR, Pearlman RA. How doctors and patients discuss routine clinical decisions. Informed decision making in the outpatient setting. *J Gen Intern Med* 1997; **12** (6): 339–45.
19. Pencheon D. Matching demand and supply fairly and efficiently. *BMJ* 1998; **316** (7145): 1665–7.
20. President's Commission for the Study of Ethical Problems in Medicine and Biomedical and Behavioral Research. Making Health Care Decisions: A Report on the Ethical and Legal Implications of Informed Consent in the Patient–Practitioner Relationship. US Government Printing Office: Washington, DC, 1982.
21. Katz J. *The Silent World of Doctor and Patient*. Free Press: New York, 1984.
22. Kasper JF, Mulley AG, Wennberg JE. Developing shared decision-making programs to improve the quality of health care. *Qual Rev Bull* 1992; **12**: 183–90.
23. Coulter A, Entwistle V, Gilbert D. Sharing decisions with patients: is the information good enough? *BMJ* 1999; **318**: 318–22.
24. Towle A, Godolphin W. Framework for teaching and learning informed shared decision making. *BMJ* 1999; **319**: 766–71.
25. Coulter A. Paternalism or partnership? Patients have grown up-and there's no going back. Editorial. *BMJ* 1999; **319** (7212): 719–20.
26. Guadagnoli E, Ward P. Patient participation in decision-making. *Soc Sci Med* 1998; **47** (3): 329–39.
27. Charles C, Redko C, Whelan T, Gafni A, Reyno L. Doing nothing is no choice: lay constructions of treatment decision-making among women with early-stage breast cancer. *Sociol Health Illness* 1998; **20**: 71–95.

11

Ethical Values in the Treatment of Depression and Anxiety

JOHN LILJA[1], SAM LARSSON[2], DAVID HAMILTON[3] AND
MIA BAUER[4]

[1]Department of Biochemistry and Pharmacy, Abo Academy University,
Turku, Finland [2]Department of Social Work, University of Stockholm and
Karolinska Institute, Center for Dependency Disorders, Magnus Huss Clinic,
Stockholm, Sweden [3]Department of Adult and Continuing Education,
University of Glasgow, Glasgow, UK [4]Statoil, Bergen, Norway

ABSTRACT

In any analysis of depression and anxiety these conditions can be viewed
from several different perspectives. In this chapter we restrict our analysis
to four different perspectives: biological, interactional, flow and symptom.
The selection of any of the four has a number of implications in terms of the
recommended type of treatment, treatment goals and the ways in which it is
determined whether or not these goals have been achieved.

The four perspectives are often combined. However, it is necessary to
look at the perspectives individually if our task is to analyse how prescribers
and patients combine the different perspectives.

There has been intensive debate about the new antidepressants. Arguments
and counter arguments reflect different ethical values regarding depression
and anxiety. For those who have a restrictive attitude to the use of drugs,
personal difficulties like divorce or the death of a family member should be
handled by psychosocial coping strategies. The main counter argument is that

Pharmaceutical Ethics. Edited by S. Salek and A. Edgar.
© 2002 John Wiley & Sons, Ltd.

the new antidepressants can allow formerly inhibited people to exercise power in social areas. Also, there is a value conflict on a theoretical and philosophical level. The materialists, like most of those who subscribe to a biological perspective, argue that mental processes can be reduced to brain processes. Chemical substances affect the brain and so the mental processes can also be changed. This lends a positive attitude to the use of psychotropics for depression and anxiety. On the other hand, interactionists argue that traumatic events, e.g. during childhood, can be memorized in the cognitive system and can also affect the body, e.g. causing symptoms of depression. For interactionists, psychotropics are much less important because the drug is normally not assumed to influence the individual's governing self.

General practitioners (GPs) detect only about half of their patients who have a depressive disorder as identified by a clinical symptom scale. However, they tend to diagnose correctly almost all of the patients with psychological symptoms. It is probably difficult to teach GPs to detect depressed patients who present with sleeping problems. If this view is accepted there is a great need for clinical trials involving the kind of depressed patient whom GPs encounter. In such trials different GP communication strategies alone or in combination with pharmacological treatment have to be compared to find which strategy is most effective in reducing symptoms of depression and anxiety.

Our knowledge of those factors that determine the prognosis for a patient suffering from clinical depression or anxiety is so rudimentary that reliable pharmacoeconomic calculations which aim to compare pharmacological therapy with non-pharmacological therapy cannot be made.

To conclude:

- Therapists ought to provide their patients with information about different perspectives on depression and anxiety. It is unethical for a therapist to restrict herself to only one perspective when talking with a patient.
- In research different perspectives on depression and anxiety ought to be combined. We need to know when and how to use pharmacological and sociopsychological treatments in primary care.
- We need to develop and evaluate effective communication strategies for primary health care professionals. At present little help is available to such professionals in selecting communication strategies for their patients with depression and anxiety.

THE ISSUE

Today ethical values in medicine and pharmacy can mean two different things: firstly, how they influence and ought to influence the individual patient–professional interaction and secondly, how they influence and ought to influence organizations in health care. Often authors concentrate upon the first of these meanings. However, we shall give consideration to both meanings in this chapter.

Further, we shall discuss not only explicit values but also those values that are implicit or hidden in what we shall call "perspectives" and "dimensions in evaluations". By this we mean frames of reference which include sets of concepts used in the analysis of the phenomenon under discussion. It seems to be characteristic both of medicine and of pharmacy to keep many of their values implicit and hidden.

Traditionally, in the language of health professionals, the assessments and decisions taken in clinical practice were regarded in neutral terms, as reflecting professional values which were not possible to transfer to explicit public values. However, some problems, e.g. how to prescribe and use psychotropics, have become public issues. When this has happened the values are often formulated in more explicit terms. This clarification of ethical values is normally not done in scientific articles. Rather, it is in popular books that the opposing views of this problem are published, and it is there that a number of professionals present their standpoints. The books by Kramer and Breggin which constitute part of the antidepressant debate (1–3) are recent examples which have made ethical values in this area of medicine much more clear (see the discussion which follows).

Thomas Kuhn suggested that only one perspective has a dominant position at any specific time in a profession (4). Every so often the efforts of a new generation of researchers result in that dominant perspective being forced aside to make way for its successor. However, what is now happening in the field of psychotropics is that Kuhn's proposition no longer holds sway. It seems that a number of perspectives can exist side by side at the same time in the field of psychotropics. No more is it the case that health professionals have one perspective and the general public another. Instead we find a spectrum of different perspectives within medicine as well as among the general public. Also, as will be described in this chapter, similar perspectives can be observed among health professionals and among lay people. Differences in the perspectives held can be found within each group as well as between the groups.

THE ACTOR–SPECTATOR PARADOX

Before analysing the perspectives concerning psychotropics we must first describe a model detailing how the position of the actor determines the perspective. This model is called the actor–spectator paradox and is shown in Figure 11.1 (5, pp. 71–85). It is an empirical model which says that

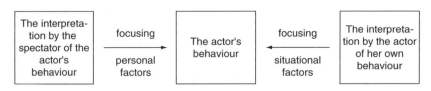

Figure 11.1 The actor–Spectator paradox

observers and actors tend to have divergent perspectives when explaining a specific behaviour. The observer (the spectator) tends to classify the behaviour of the actor according to what the observer believes the actor's intentions or characteristics are. This means that the observer makes assumptions about these aspects of the actor. However, actors tend to attribute their actions to situational requirements and not to their intentions or personalities. The observer and the actor often have quite different views about the actor's behaviour. We can say they are living in different worlds.

The actor–spectator paradigm can be applied when analysing how a practising GP meets a patient with symptoms of depression and anxiety. The GP observes the patient's behaviour and based on her observations makes assumptions about the patient's condition and what has caused that condition (this will be discussed more later). The patient may have a different view about her condition and the reasons for it. However, an empathic GP tries to understand the patient's view of her condition. This is necessary for the communication to be effective and to ensure patient compliance. Patient and GP have to come up with an agreement as to which therapy to select. Of course, GPs vary in their capacities to be empathic and in achieving a realistic understanding of their patients' emotions, cognitions and situations as their patients see these (6).

The GP will probably reach an understanding of her patient's views on some level. Nevertheless, there will remain a difference between them. The dependency controversy provides one illustration of one such remaining difference between the views of a GP and of her patient. According to most GPs, psychotropic dependency is often defined as the presence of severe withdrawal problems when stopping taking a drug. This means that most GPs do not regard antidepressants as a class of drugs which cause dependency, because these drugs seldom cause significant withdrawal problems. However, many patients define drug dependency in another way. They often define dependency according to their own perception of the difficulty they have in stopping taking a psychotropic. According to this definition antidepressants can be viewed as a dependency-forming class of drugs. A patient can think of herself as hooked on drug use because although she wants to stop taking the drug she cannot do so. However, from her GP's point of view, this may not be seen as dependency because this class of drugs seldom produces significant withdrawal reactions (7, p. 242).

However, the actor–spectator model should not lead us to the belief that all differences in perspectives are caused by differences in professional position.

THE VALUE BASIS OF THIS CHAPTER

History can help us to understand how public values have changed in recent decades. At the start of the twentieth century health care therapy could be said to be based on the idea of "the passive patient". This meant that a patient who became ill would contact a health care professional, e.g. a physician or a pharmacist. The medical decisions were taken by the professionals while the patient was expected to concentrate on complying with the medical instructions. It was assumed that the professionals and their patients had a common goal, to cure the patient.

From the 1970s onwards a new health care ideology developed. According to this new ideology a member of the public is expected to rely upon her own initiative to look after her health. The patient has a right to open, honest and detailed information about her medical condition and available treatment options. Further, it is ethically important that patients should be encouraged to ask questions and to learn about different therapeutic options. The patient's own values and attitudes have to be respected and the patient must be given the opportunity to select from similar therapeutic options. All these rights of the patient can be summed up in the "informed consent" requirements (see discussion below).

Professional groups seem to have lost the dominant position they had at the beginning of the century. A number of new, well-organized bodies have entered the scene and argued that they have legitimate rights to influence medical decision-making, e.g. political bodies, financial institutions, insurance companies, patient/consumer organizations. This means that the experts no longer have unquestioned authority in their own field. They now are expected more and more to be responsible for collecting valid data about a specific problem, analysing the data and making the data and their analysis public. This changed role, however, has not ensured that in the eyes of the general public an expert's conclusions are always valid.

DIFFERENT PERSPECTIVES ON DEPRESSION AND ANXIETY

In any analysis of depression and anxiety these conditions can be viewed from several different perspectives (8). Here for pedagogical reasons we are restricting our analysis to four different perspectives. The selection of any of the four has a number of implications in terms of the recommended type of treatment, treatment goals and the ways in which it is determined whether or not these goals have been achieved. However, regardless of which perspective is employed, a reduction in the severity of the patient's symptoms must surely be one of the treatment goals. Depending on which perspective is chosen, other treatment goals can be used side by side with a reduction in the patient's symptoms.

The four perspectives are as follows.

1. Depression and anxiety are caused by dysfunctional biochemical processes. This perspective is often called the "biological perspective". At least some of the people who apply this perspective think genetic factors play an important role in determining an individual's vulnerability. A doctor who has this perspective often recommends pharmacological treatment for patients who fulfil the criteria for depression or anxiety disorders. For example, by taking antidepressant drugs the patient's biochemical processes are expected to become more functional and the corresponding symptoms of depression are expected to decrease. Among psychiatrists such a biological perspective seems common (9).

Representatives of the biological perspective often measure results by the level of the dysfunctional symptoms present (see perspective 4 below). However, treatment results can be measured in two different ways. One way is to say that the treatment can be viewed as effective if the symptoms, as measured by a symptom index, have been reduced by 50% or more. The other way is to argue that it is an effective therapy if the symptoms when treated and when measured by an accepted psychiatric scale (in practice the DSM, i.e. "The Diagnostic and Statistical Manual of Mental Disorders" published by the American Psychiatric Association, or the ICD, i.e. "International Classification of Diseases") no longer fulfil the criteria for the psychiatric condition. This means that a treatment can be effective according to the first meaning but not according to the second meaning or vice versa.

The biological perspective encourages the belief that a rather short-term evaluation, e.g. over six to eight weeks, gives valuable information. In such a brief time span it is possible to determine if the biochemical processes of the individual can be returned to near normal levels. Why we have so few long-term evaluations of psychotropic drugs is partly determined by an acceptance of this perspective. Another reason is the costs in terms of money and time of long-term evaluations.

2. Depression and anxiety are caused by an interaction between an individual's internal cognitive system and the demands of the indivi-

dual's situation. This can be called the "interactional perspective". Those who adhere to the interactional perspective tend to believe that the outcome cannot be evaluated by the presence (or absence) of the symptoms alone. Also, according to this view, we have to wait longer than a few months to see if the individual has recovered or not.

The interactional perspective can be further divided into situational orientation and, secondly, cognitive and emotional orientation. Those who subscribe to situational orientation think that environmental factors, e.g. mourning, are the main causes of a patient's symptoms. A positive attitude towards situational orientation seems to be common among GPs (9,10). Also, the general public tends to regard depression and anxiety as being caused by environmental or situational factors, e.g. conflict at work, disputes in the family setting (11). Counselling about practical and daily matters is a treatment often recommended by those who have this situational orientation. We can expect a GP with such a perspective to encourage discussions about what has happened and about what can be done to help the patient to recover. Also, the recommended treatment often combines a situational orientation with the energy perspective discussed below. For example, to get a person in a state of mild depression to take part in social and other activities is often seen by the general public as beneficial to the individual concerned (11–13).

Supporters of the situational orientation approach tend when evaluating treatment to combine an analysis of the dysfunctional symptom levels with a consideration of how the patient has improved socially. According to this perspective a relapse is seen as much in terms of social functioning as in terms of symptoms.

The second type of interactional perspective can be called "cognitive and emotional orientation" and includes identity factors as causes of depression and anxiety. Here the therapist's interest is focused on the patient's inner world and not the outer world as in the situational orientation. Those who have a cognitive and an emotional orientation regard the patient's dysfunctional cognitive system as the main explanation for the disorder. Here, cognitive therapy is often a recommended treatment strategy for depressive or anxiety disorders, e.g. (14).

The psychodynamic framework focuses upon the interaction between the individual and her environment and how the personality develops during childhood. However, both the psychodynamic and the cognitive frameworks include cognitive and emotional factors. Also, both frameworks take into account unconscious influences upon these cognitive and emotional factors (15).

For those who have a cognitive and emotional orientation treatment is often assessed by combining an analysis of the dysfunctional symptoms with a study of how the selection of psychological coping strategies has improved during the treatment period.

People who have an interactional perspective do not necessarily see symptoms like agitation or sadness as something bad. Instead the symptoms may help the individual to reconstruct her cognitions and develop a better fit between her cognitions and her environment. The symptoms could be a starting point for "personal growth" (16).

In the interactional perspective the relationship between the therapist and the patient is very important. A "therapeutic alliance" including psychological warmth, trust and empathy will increase the patient's willingness to search for new cognitions and new relationships with her environment (17,18). Through an empathic understanding the therapist can achieve a relationship of trust with her patient. However, if the patient really wants a psychotropic and suffers severe depression or anxiety, perhaps even of an episodic nature, a GP might prescribe a psychotropic as a way of building up a trusting relationship.

3. Depression and anxiety are disorders where the individual can no longer control her psychic energy. From this perspective loss of capacity to control one's own energy leads to affective symptoms because energy control is necessary to achieve desired emotional states such as satisfaction and happiness. In the phenomenological tradition these states are called "flows" and are characterized by individual, goal-directed activities where the individual loses her sense of time, sees the activity as of value in itself and becomes free from worries (8,19). According to Csikszentmihalyi (19), a state of "flow" is when: "Your mind isn't wandering, you are not thinking of something else; you are totally involved with what you are doing. Your energy is flowing very smoothly. You feel relaxed, comfortable and energetic".

However, when a person is depressed there are often inner turmoils and crises which occupy her internal world. To be free of anxiety and depression it is necessary, according to Csikszentmihalyi, to make oneself free of the demands of the situation in order to experience flow.

This perspective may be called "the flow perspective" and it is possible to combine it with perspectives 1 and 2 above. The reason is that this perspective "explains" depression and on a lower level is much closer to the symptoms experienced. This means an incapacity to experience flow can be caused both by biochemical and cognitive factors.

In a therapy based on a flow perspective the patient has to be helped to break her negative thought patterns, inner turmoils and cognitive incongruences. This will help her to focus her awareness on what she regards as an interesting task. This can be expected to facilitate the achievement of flow.

4. Depression and anxiety are a number of specified dysfunctional symptoms analysed in a defined way. This is the perspective of the DSM scheme that is often recommended by medics. The alternative ICD scheme of psychiatric classification is more often used in Europe and is based on the same perspective. In the definitions of major depression and generalized anxiety the causal factors are disregarded in these schemes. The reason for this is that the application of causal factors diminishes the reliability when diagnosing a specific patient as having a psychiatric condition. If a diagnostician has to base her diagnosis on assumed causal factors we would have much lower reliability than in a diagnostic system, where the causal factors are ignored. By basing the diagnostic system on symptoms whose reliability is accepted, a comparatively high level of reliability in the ultimate diagnosis can be achieved.

However, to our knowledge GPs avoid the DSM and the ICD systems because of their complexity. Another reason for their lack of popularity among GPs is that they need aetiological models when assessing, treating and communicating with patients suffering from depression and anxiety (see discussion below).

COMBINATIONS OF PERSPECTIVES

The four perspectives described above are often combined. For example, an empathic and concerned GP tends to begin her discussion with a patient with symptoms of depression and/or anxiety by investigating the patient's environmental stresses (a situational orientation). At subsequent meetings the physician is likely to look at the cognitions the patient has (a cognitive and emotional orientation). To begin to discuss the patient's cognitions at the first meeting could be disastrous to the patient's self-confidence. Also, trying to alter the patient's cognitions requires that a trusting relationship has been established. If a change in the symptoms cannot be observed after a number of meetings with the patient the GP might prescribe an antidepressant (the GP here would be taking a biological perspective). Later the GP might try to follow the recovery process by analysing the patient's symptoms (a symptom perspective), social functioning (a situational orientation) and psychological coping strategies (a cognitive and emotional orientation).

So if people try to combine the four perspectives what is the reason for describing them separately? We think it necessary to look at the perspectives individually because the crucial question is not whether people combine the perspectives or not. Rather, the most interesting issue is analysing *how* prescribers combine the perspectives when diagnosing and treating depression and anxiety. We think different GPs combine the perspectives in different ways. How an empathic GP might combine the perspectives has already been described. One interesting research task for the future would be to identify how frequently GPs adopt a combined approach such as described above. Perhaps, thereafter, an education programme could be designed to encourage GPs to adopt a more empathic combination of perspectives.

THE DEBATE ABOUT THE VALUE OF
ANTIDEPRESSANT DRUGS

Whether a GP prescribes a psychotropic is influenced by her views on the advantages and disadvantages of antidepressants and anxiolytic drugs. It is well known from a number of studies that attitudes to psychotropics vary among GPs and influence their prescribing of such medication (20–22). Table 11.1 gives a summary of the most frequent criticisms and counter arguments in the antidepressant debate. Some of the points of criticism are more strongly connected to ethical values than others. For example, the first point of criticism, that antidepressants are overused, is linked with views about how people should handle their difficulties. Those critical tend to support the view that personal difficulties, like a divorce or a death of a family member, should be handled by psychosocial coping strategies, e.g. social contacts, identity changes. Of course, such a value norm can be supported by empirical hypotheses and deductions from future situations. For example, the restrictive attitude to antidepressants could be supported by a prognosis of what will happen if all our negative emotions can be avoided by the use of drugs. This would lead to a completely different society where most people would take psychotropics almost on a daily basis. For those who have a restrictive attitude towards drugs such a future is abhorrent.

Table 11.1   A summary of the antidepressant debate

Critical argument	Counter argument
1. Antidepressants tend to be overused (2, pp. 194–212)	1. Antidepressants tend to be underused (1, p. 274)
2. Side-effects are significant (2, pp. 199–207)	2. New antidepressants have few side-effects (1, pp. 301–13)
3. Antidepressants reduce the patient's emotional responsiveness (2, p. 208)	3. New antidepressants allow formerly inhibited people to exercise power in social and political areas that previously made them uncomfortable (1, p. 272)
4. We do not know the effects of long-term use (2, p. 207)	4. New antidepressants increase the patient's autonomy (1, p. 265)
5. Prozac can be regarded as a stimulant associated with considerable withdrawal problems (3)	5. Prozac is associated with few withdrawal problems (1)

However, those who have a less restrictive attitude to drug therapy and perhaps see antidepressants as a blessing for those who need them also have arguments to back their value norm. They often say that anti-depressants have been shown to be effective, i.e. they decrease the dysfunctional symptoms and have only a few side-effects and a few withdrawal symptoms. This proposition seems to rely solely on factual empirical evidence but, of course, it is based upon values. First, as discussed above, to restrict the evaluation to the measurement of symptoms is a value statement. Second, data about side-effects has to be interpreted in value terms before the data can be used in decision-making (23). Some people will accept the side-effects of an antidepressant in a specific situation while other people will not because they may see other ways of dealing with the situation. Third, as has been explained in detail by Breggin et al. (3), what withdrawal symptoms are cannot be decided without a conceptual model which helps us to determine if a symptom is a withdrawal symptom or not. If we include minor symptoms among withdrawal symptoms, like difficulties in achieving flow without an antidepressant after being used to it, then we cannot argue that Prozac has few withdrawal effects. According to Breggin's withdrawal model Prozac could be classified as a stimulant. However, this is not what people with other withdrawal models will say.

The debate about psychotropics has also taken place on a more theoretical and philosophical level. It is possible to distinguish between two different perspectives of the relationship between mind and brain, a materialistic versus an interactionist perspective (24–27). These two perspectives tend to be associated with different attitudes to the use of psychotropics:

1. The materialist's perspective: A parallelism between brain and mind is assumed. According to this perspective mental processes are almost identical to, or can be reduced to, brain processes. These are to a large extent assumed to be determined by genetic factors. An individual who has a materialistic perspective may, we argue, more easily adopt a positive attitude to psychotropics. By using chemical substances that affect the brain, the mental processes can also be influenced. According to most materialists healthy individuals have one personality only. People with personality problems can be helped by drugs to achieve a more functional daily lifestyle.

2. The interactionist's perspective: Here, mental processes and the development of the person are seen as the result of an interaction between the individual and her environment. Traumatic events, e.g. during childhood, can be memorized in the cognitive system and may lead to negative psychosomatic or psychological symptoms. However, traumatic events are assumed to affect both the mental processes and the brain processes at the same time. Also, there is an interaction between the mind and the brain.

Brain processes influence the mental processes, e.g. as a result of genetic factors, but the reverse is also the case.

Today it is popular to assume that an individual may have a number of different "small minds" or identities. The individual may switch between her "small minds" with the aid of a governing self depending on the situation the individual is facing (28). The individual may experience one identity while taking a psychotropic and another identity when not taking the drug. The governing self is in general assumed not to be affected by the psychotropic used. A long-term user of a psychotropic might find that her non-psychotropic identities are underdeveloped. To reduce dependency on the psychotropic the patient needs to develop a whole new set of "small minds", which can require considerable effort in terms of time and psychic energy. This means that the use of chemical substances is much less important for most interactionists than for materialists. Thus, interactionists tend to have a restrictive attitude to psychotropic prescribing.

HOW A COMBINATION OF DIMENSIONS IN THE ANALYSIS OF THERAPIES WOULD INFLUENCE THE WAY DRUG CLINICAL TRIALS ARE DESIGNED

Practically no clinical trial of drugs in this field is based on pharmacological treatment alone. In almost all clinical trials pharmacological treatment is combined with psychological counselling. This means that in clinical trials we need to combine the perspectives discussed above. Not only the severity and frequency of symptoms but also improvements in coping strategies, self-confidence and social activities should be included as outcome measures in clinical trials. To understand how the patient is affected by negative events and difficulties during treatment, "life event scales" ought to be used before and during treatment in clinical trials (29).

The relationship between pharmacological treatment and patient social learning ought to be analysed. The main question here is to understand when and how a pharmacological treatment can facilitate patient learning of new coping strategies and under which circumstances such a treatment can be a barrier to patient learning. For example, elderly patients might decide not to learn other coping behaviours while receiving pharmacological treatment, whereas a group of younger patients might use the more positive emotional level as a starting point for identifying such supportive techniques. Also, whether the patient will search for psychological coping strategies while receiving pharmacological treatment might depend on which cognitive models are offered by the GP and the cognitive and social resources of the patient.

A major problem is that so few clinical trials in primary care are undertaken. One reason is said to be that such trials are impractical because the placebo-treated group has such a high recovery rate that it is difficult to record any differences between the placebo group and the experimental group who receive an active drug (29). This, to us, does not seem an acceptable argument because the great majority of those suffering from depression are seen in primary health care.

What is important is to analyse how a group of primary care patients with specific characteristics, e.g. symptoms, social capacity, social resources, coping strategies, sense of meaning, self-confidence and the events and difficulties they have experienced or experience at the start of the study, will recover in terms of symptoms, social capacity, social resources, coping strategies, sense of meaning and self-confidence. The treatment period should be long enough to make it possible to see changes in these variables (29).

WHY DO GPS NOT DETECT PATIENTS WITH DEPRESSION IN THE FREQUENCY INDICATED BY EPIDEMIOLOGICAL OR DIAGNOSTIC MEASURES?

There are a great number of studies indicating GPs in their practice do not identify all the cases identified by diagnostic schemes. For example, in a study by Ormel et al. (30) GPs identified only 56% of the new cases identified by the Present State Examination clinical interviewing scheme (PSE, which applies the ICD criteria to classify psychiatric disorders) as having depression or anxiety.

One reason why GPs do not detect cases of depression and anxiety is that most patients make health care contact because of sleeping difficulties and expect the GP to deal with these complaints. Also, some GPs do not regard it as their duty to treat depression and anxiety in patients who do not ask for help for such problems (31, pp. 167–172).

In a number of studies it has been found that patients who mentioned that they think they are depressed and/or anxious or have other evident psychological symptoms are far more likely to be identified by GPs as cases of depression and/or anxiety than patients presenting with somatic symptoms (10,30,32–35). Also, the nature of communication during the encounter influences the probability of the GP detecting affective symptoms (36, p. 101; 37, pp. 75–81; 38).

These types of studies have their shortcomings. For example, in the Ormel et al. study (30), the PSE scheme identified the cases with depression or anxiety by assessing patients' symptoms, while the GPs were asked to assess whether a patient had a specific psychiatric disorder or symptoms due to psychological problems or stress. This means that the perspectives are quite different. The PSE scheme is entirely based upon symptoms while the GPs were asked to make their assessments on an environmental causal analysis. This way of assessing a case is, of course, based on a tradition found among GPs in clinical practice. GPs do take causal factors into account when they assess whether or not a patient is suffering from depression or anxiety or not. Because of the differences in perspective a 100% agreement would be most unlikely.

It is generally accepted by experts that efforts should be made to get GPs to identify (and diagnose) more patients with depression and anxiety. Some publications support the view that GPs are thought to underestimate the number of patients with depression, e.g. NIH Consensus Conference on Late Life (39). However, according to the Ormel et al. study (30), GPs do not underestimate patients with psychological problems and stress but they do not identify all cases which, according to the symptom scales, have what we would call depression and anxiety. An evaluation of those cases which are overlooked will be discussed in the next part of this chapter.

IS IT AN ADVANTAGE IF DEPRESSION OR ANXIETY DISORDERS ARE DETECTED BY GPS?

As discussed above some expert groups are very eager to stress how important it is that GPs detect depression and anxiety disorders. Implicit in this is the notion that more patients should be prescribed antidepressants (39).

In only a few studies has the aim been to collect data about the social costs of undetected patients. In the study by Ormel et al. (30) it was found that the prognosis was much better for those patients who were detected by GPs compared with those who went undetected but were, nevertheless, depression/anxiety cases according to the PSE. The Ormel et al. study went further by presenting data explaining why the detected cases had a more positive prognosis. The main reason was not that the detected cases were prescribed psychotropics more often. More than half of the non-severe detected cases were not given a drug but still had a more positive outcome than the non-severe non-detected cases. The explanation for this was that the GPs tended to pick up those cases which had mainly psychological symptoms, and avoided patients with mainly somatic symptoms indicating depression. The former group had a much more positive outcome than the latter. This means that a sampling bias of the GPs is one reason why detected cases have a more positive outcome than undetected cases. The authors also suggest that it might be simpler for GPs to help patients with psychological symptoms to recover from their depression than patients having mainly somatic depressive symptoms (30). This is because it can be expected to be easier for

GPs to act upon a patient's sociopsychological problems if the patient from the start accepts that she has such problems. The GPs could then discuss the treatment with her in terms of sociopsychological models, e.g. an interactional or energy perspective as discussed above.

This means that the difficulty is to get the non-detected cases to formulate their problems in psychological terms. If the GP is able to do this, the patient might get a more positive result measured in terms of a reduction in her symptoms of depression and anxiety. So the policy implication is perhaps not to encourage more prescribing of psychotropics, but to improve communication skills among GPs.

HOW TO ANALYSE THE THERAPY PROVIDED BY GPS FOR PATIENTS WITH DEPRESSION AND ANXIETY SYMPTOMS

In a great number of pharmacoepidemiological studies, the association between the age, sex and socioeconomic characteristics of the patient and psychotropic prescribing have been analysed. Also, there are a number of studies investigating how age, education, specialization and attitudes of the physician are associated with psychotropic prescribing behaviour. However, in these studies the researchers have not analysed the cognitive processes of the physician when she decides to prescribe a psychotropic or not.

Also, in analysing how GPs choose treatments for patients with symptoms of depression and anxiety it is necessary to combine an analysis of the drug prescribed with an analysis of the communication taking place during the encounter. There are both empirical and theoretical reasons for such a combined research strategy. The empirical reason is that a combination of pharmacological and counselling therapy in primary care might lead to better results than one of the treatment strategies alone (31). The theoretical reason is that beneficial long-term results from pharmacological treatment are very much dependent on the psychological coping strategies the patient develops during that kind of treatment. Of course the patient cannot develop new coping strategies on her own. These must normally be developed by interaction with people in the patient's social network. However, the GP might promote and facilitate the adoption of new coping strategies and the making of new contacts. The GP can encourage the patient to make contact with relatives, to engage in physical activities and to join social organizations. This means that it is an advantage if the GP keeps in mind all the perspectives discussed above during the treatment.

There is wide variation in how GPs assess a video-vignette showing a patient with symptoms of depression and anxiety (40,41). For example, a physician who has a biological orientation tends to be much more optimistic about the outcome of treatment for depression and anxiety than a colleague who has a more psychological orientation. The former often recommends psychotropics and believes that these drugs help the patient in the short term without too much effort by the patient on her own behalf. Physicians who are more psychologically oriented tend to think that recovery processes are much more complex and take considerable effort and time (42). This means that these groups have different time perspectives and different ways of judging outcome.

We believe there are five main dimensions involved in a GP's assessment as to whether a patient should be prescribed a psychotropic when the patient shows symptoms of depression or anxiety.

1. The GP's assessment of the level of severity of the symptoms and the social effects these symptoms have.

The more severe the symptoms and the more severe the social consequences, the greater the likelihood that a psychotropic will be prescribed, e.g. (30,43,44).

In a study by two of the authors it was noted that this type of assessment can be influenced by continuing education on a three-day course. It was found that health professionals assessed a number of video patients as having much milder symptoms after the course than before (45). The reason was probably that on the course they learned that treatment by counselling could achieve good results. The results could be explained by a cognitive dissonance model. Previously health professionals were forced to think of the cases as serious because they saw few options to prescribing a psychotropic. After the course they were aware of other treatment options. They did not feel forced to prescribe a psychotropic. So, in effect, many cases were regarded as much milder.

2. The GP's assumptions regarding the reasons for the patient's condition.

Traditionally someone with endogenous depression was more likely to receive an antidepressant than a patient with evident exogenous depression caused by environmental factors, e.g. mourning. Even if the endogenous–exogenous dichotomy is not used very much today, we think such assessments influence the probability of prescribing psychotropics.

The assessment of the causal factor for the depressive disorder may influence the assessment of the severity of the symptoms. If the depression can be "explained" in terms of a negative event, people (physicians and the general public) tend to regard the depressive episode as less serious than if the episode cannot be explained by an environmental factor (29).

3. The GP's assumptions regarding the patient's prognosis with or without an antidepressant.

We can expect that GPs make assumptions regarding a patient's cognitive and social resources and use these assumptions as the basis for their analysis of the likelihood of a reasonable recovery with or without psychotropic use. If the patient has sufficient cognitive and social resources at her disposal we can expect the GP to treat her by counselling and decide against prescribing an antidepressant or an anxiolytic drug.

Of course, the patient's prognosis is associated with the severity of her symptoms. Severe symptoms are often associated with a more negative prognosis, e.g. (46–48). However, the prognosis is very much dependent on the length of time the patient has suffered from her symptoms. If the patient has experienced her symptoms over a long period or had earlier episodes of the disorder we can expect the recovery process to be much slower than for a patient who has had symptoms over a short while (42,49). Also, elderly depressive patients tend to have a more negative prognosis than younger patients with the same severity of symptoms (50).

4. The GP's assumptions regarding the treatment preferences of the patient.

We can expect the GP to be more willing to prescribe an antidepressant if she thinks that the patient wants an antidepressant than if no such wish is indicated by the patient (51,52). One reason is that the GP wants to meet the patient's requests as far as possible. Another reason is that the GP sees little sense in prescribing for a patient who will not comply with the treatment. Also, there is a strong tendency for GPs to continue prescribing a psychotropic if the patient is satisfied and wants this. GPs seldom get into arguments with patients about them stopping taking psychotropics (53,54).

In the professional literature there is a debate about the role of the patient's values. Some argue that the rule should be that all patients satisfying the criteria for major depression should be persuaded to take an antidepressant. Others insist that the patient should be encouraged to influence the treatment strategy. A patient with mild or medium severe depression should be given the right to decide for herself whether to take an antidepressant or not, without any effort being made to affect her decision. Also, according to this latter standpoint, only patients with severe depression should be encouraged to take an antidepressant in combination with non-pharmacological treatments (55). This is supported by the empirical evidence, which indicates that a combination of pharmacological therapy and psychotherapy is more effective in the treatment of the more severe cases of major depression. However, combination therapy does not give any further advantages than psychotherapy alone in the treatment of less severe cases which fulfil the criteria for major depression, e.g. (56,57).

5. The GP's assumptions regarding the depressed patient's risk of suicide.

If the risk of suicide is high we can expect the GP to prescribe an antidepressant (58).

With better outcome studies combined with more surveys of the cognitive processes by which GPs in practice prescribe (to video patients or real-life patients), we shall be more favourably placed to plan continuing education courses for health and social professionals on how to treat depression and anxiety, because we should be able to identify desired cognitive processes among the prescribers.

FREEDOM OF INFORMATION

At the beginning of the twentieth century, when the passive patient was accepted as the norm, medical data and discussions of medical matters were kept secret from the general public. Because health care professionals were supposed to take all medical decisions, this restricted distribution of medical data was regarded as a legitimate procedure. According to the new active patient paradigm, patients should now take medical decisions in co-operation with the health professionals. However, the decisions ought to be based on the ethical values held by the individual patient. In practice this means that it is often not enough to provide the patient with the medical facts. Many patients also need to be provided with decision models illustrating how to take a rational decision based on the experiences of patients who have had similar conditions previously. It is an ethical obligation that patients ought to be provided with information about the different perspectives on depression and anxiety as described above, and the arguments for each perspective. However, in practice health professionals unconsciously may reveal their own attitudes to each of the perspectives. This cannot entirely be avoided even if the aim is to provide each patient with information about different perspectives and different treatment options. This can be regarded as an argument for the development of written or multimedia educational material that can complement the verbal information provided during the medical encounter.

Now the Internet, which is available to many people, gives us a huge amount of health-related information. The main problem with the information available via the Internet is that the quality varies considerably. Often no references to empirical data and empirical studies are made. This can be contrasted with the service available to professionals who can depend upon Medline or the Cochrane Library for extensive and reliable information. However, to have such sources widely available does not solve the issue of freedom of information for the general public. The information in these systems is not prepared and structured to answer the health queries and solve the medical problems of the general public.

SOME ETHICAL PROBLEMS IN PHARMACOECONOMIC STUDIES

The most evident problems in pharmacoeconomic studies can be summarized via the following points.

1. The reliability and validity of incidence and prevalence data concerning depression and anxiety are questionable. The reason is that researchers use different definitions and measurements to determine the incidence and prevalence. For example, the life prevalence for major depression varies between 2 and 20% between different studies (59).

Also, there is a significant variation in the population regarding incidence and prevalence of depression and anxiety. Some groups will have extremely low levels while others will have considerably high risks of developing these conditions.

2. It is very difficult to make a reliable prognosis for a patient suffering from depression and anxiety. In some pharmacoeconomic studies the prescriber is asked to assess the expected treatment period with or without the use of antidepressants. This is not an acceptable method because we cannot assume that physicians (or non-physicians) can make a reliable prognosis regarding the length of an episode of depression or anxiety.

The outcome of the treatment is determined by a complex combination of cognitive, environmental and biochemical factors. Also, the outcome is very much influenced by the type of counselling therapy offered, in combination with the pharmacological treatment.

3. The results of a comparison of a course of drug treatment with that of a non-drug treatment are very much dependent on the content of the non-drug treatment course.

It is not enough to describe the counselling therapy in terms of the ''school'' to which the therapist subscribes, e.g. cognitive therapy, behavioural therapy, psychodynamic therapy. We need to go much deeper and see what the therapist actually does in the course of the therapy. Further, comparison is very much dependent on how the patients have been selected. For patients with severe depression or who are experiencing a severe episode of anxiety, pharmacological therapy is often combined with counselling. For other patients, psychotherapy alone might be the best approach. The problem today is that we do not know which type of patient is most helped by pharmacological treatment.

4. How do we set values on the benefits achieved by the treatment?

To set values on an emotional state is associated with value assumptions. Even if a group of lay people is asked to establish the values, it could be argued that these values only reflect those of the group. Further, an individual may have values that deviate from those set by the group. Also, how values are set might differ from one cultural setting to another.

It is even more questionable to set monetary values on emotional states. The variation among individuals ascribing monetary values to a specific emotional state can be expected to be huge.

Such criticisms lead us to conclude that it is too early for anyone to make reliable pharmacoeconomic calculations when comparing treatment with psychotropic drugs with non-pharmacological treatment options. We simply know too little as yet about this area to have any faith in the reliability of such calculations. However, this does not mean that we are generally critical of pharmacoeconomic calculations. For example, in a number of reputable studies a tricyclic preparation has been compared to a new antidepressant. In even such a limited analysis the data available may still be sufficiently reliable to make economic calculations of significance.

ETHICAL PROBLEMS IN OTHER PARTS OF THE HEALTH CARE SECTOR THAT AFFECT THE TREATMENT OF DEPRESSION AND ANXIETY

National drug insurance systems are based on a great number of values. Here one problem is the classification of drugs and medical conditions that determine which drugs and medical conditions should be paid for by the insurance system.

Another issue is the registration control of new psychotropic substances. Today the decisions taken inside the European Union system have a strong impact on which psychotropics are to be marketed and their therapeutic indications. The European Union system will also determine how clinical trials should be set up to permit the registration of psychotropics. The present process leading to registration of a psychotropic can take place without any comparison with non-pharmacological treatment options. This policy has to be questioned. To determine if a psychotropic is medically advantageous or not we need information about the treatment results of the drug in comparison with the results from at least one non-pharmacological treatment option.

To get more information about the new drug control system in Europe we need more detailed studies about how the system is working, including the ethical values upon which the decisions are based. The system has been transformed very quickly from national control institutions to European institutions, and we know very little about how the new system operates.

IMPLICATIONS

Implications for Therapists

Therapists ought to provide their patients with information about different perspectives on depression and anxiety. In our view it is unethical for a therapist to restrict herself to only one perspective when talking with a patient. The patient has an ethical right to be provided with the different perspectives which may help her to manage her psychosocial and medical problems.

Also, the therapist has an ethical obligation to use an empathic communication strategy when interacting with the patient. This is because an empathic strategy is a prerequisite for establishing a therapeutic alliance and open communication with the patient.

Implications for Researchers

Researchers need to clarify the perspectives of the therapists, the values upon which they base their decisions and how combinations of drug and counselling treatments are determined in clinical practice.

Also, we need to know when and how to combine pharmacological and sociopsychological treatments in primary care. Today most clinical trials of psychotropics do not include important sociopsychological variables such as data about the patient's self-confidence, the events and difficulties the patient faces, her coping strategies and her social support network. We need a much better understanding of how these factors interact with drug treatment in recovery from depression and anxiety.

Further, we need to develop and evaluate effective and empathic communication strategies for primary health care professionals. Today they are provided with little help in selecting communication strategies for their patients with depression and anxiety.

REFERENCES

1. Kramer PD. *Listening to Prozac*. Penguin: New York, 1994.
2. Breggin P. *Toxic Psychiatry: Drugs and Electroconvulsive Therapy: The Truth and the Better Alternatives*. Fontana: London, 1993.
3. Breggin P et al. *Talking Back to Prozac*. St. Martin's Press: New York, 1994.
4. Kuhn T. *The Structure of Scientific Revolutions*. University of Chicago Press: Chicago, 1965.
5. Augoustinos M et al. *Social Cognition: An Integrated Introduction*. Sage: London, 1995.
6. Mishler EG. *The Discourse of Medicine*. Ablex Publishing: Norwood, NJ, 1984.
7. Lilja J, Larsson S, Hamilton D. *Drug Communication: How Cognitive Science Can Help the Health Professionals*. Kuopio University: Kuopio, 1996.
8. Stevens R et al. The reflexive self: an experiential perspective. In *Understanding the Self*, Stevens R (ed). Sage: London, 1996; 147–218.
9. Kerr M et al. General practitioners and psychiatrists: comparison of attitudes to depression using depression attitude questionnaire. *Br J Gen Prac* 1995; **45**: 89–92.
10. Blacker SVR et al. Depressive disorder in primary care. *Br J Psychiatry* 1987; **150**: 737–51.
11. Bauer M et al. The depressive symptoms of people living in Aland and how they handle their symptoms. In press (in Swedish).
12. Rippere V. What's the thing to do when you're feeling depressed?—A pilot study. *Beh Res Ther* 1977; **15**: 185–91.
13. Parker GB et al. Coping behaviours that mediate between life events and depression. *Arch Gen Psychiatry* 1982; **39**: 1386–91.
14. Beck AT. *Depression: Clinical, Experimental and Theoretical Aspects*. Staples Press: London, 1969.
15. Eagle MN. The psychoanalytical and the cognitive unconsciousness. In *Theories of the Unconscious and Theories of the Self*, Stern R (ed). The Analytic Press: Hillsdale, NJ, 1987; 155–90.
16. Gut E. *Getting Depressed: Its Function and Failures*. Routledge: New York, 1989.
17. Rogers CR. The necessary and sufficient conditions of therapeutic personality change. *J Consult Psychol* 1957; **21**: 95–103.
18. Wheeler S. Achieving and maintaining competence. In *The Needs of Counselors and Psychotherapists*, Horton I et al. (eds). Sage: London, 1996; 120–34.
19. Csikszentmihalyi M. *Flow: The Psychology of Optimal Experience*. Harper Collins: New York, 1990.
20. Linn LS. Physician characteristics and attitudes toward legitimate use of psychotropic drugs. *J Health Soc Behav* 1971; **12**: 132–40.
21. Johnson J et al. Service utilization and social morbidity associated with depressive symptoms in the community. *JAMA* 1992; **267**: 1478–83.
22. Sorvaniemi M et al. Recognition and management of major depression in psychiatric outpatient care: a questionnaire survey. *J Affect Disord* 1996; **41**: 223–7.
23. Day JC et al. A comparison of patients' and prescribers' beliefs about neuroleptic side-effects: prevalence, distress and causation. *Acta Psychiatr Scand* 1998; **97**: 93–7.
24. Popper KR et al. *The Self and its Brain*. Springer: New York, 1977.
25. Eccles J. The human brain and the human person. In *Main and Brain*, Eccles J (ed). Paragon: New York, 1987; 85–102.

26. Eccles J. Cerebral activity and the freedom of the will. In *Main and Brain*, Eccles J (ed). Paragon: New York, 1987; 159–84.
27. Eccles J. *Evolution of the Brain—Creation of the Self*. Routledge: London/New York, 1991.
28. Ornstein R. *Multimind*. Macmillan: London, 1986.
29. Klerman GL et al. Evaluating drug treatments of depressive disorders. In *Clinical Evaluation of Psychotropic Drugs*, Prien RF et al. (eds). Raven Press: New York, 1994; 281–325.
30. Ormel J et al. Recognition, management and outcome of psychological disorders in primary care: a naturalistic follow-up study. *Psychol Med* 1990; **20**: 909–23.
31. Lilja J, Larsson S. New Perspectives on Depression and Anxiety. Folkhalsoinstitutet, Stockholm, 1998 (in Swedish).
32. Clare AW et al. Some problems affecting the diagnosis and classification of depressive disorders in primary care. In *Mental Illness in Primary Care*, Shepherd M et al. (eds). Tavistock Publishing: London/New York, 1986; 7–26.
33. Katon W et al. Depression and chronic medical illness. *J Clin Psychiatry* 1990; **51** (Suppl 6); 3–11.
34. Kirmayer LJ et al. Somatization and the recognition of depression and anxiety in primary care. *Am J Psychiatry* 1993; **150**: 734–41.
35. Katon W et al. A randomized trial of psychiatric consultation with distressed high utilizers. *Gen Hosp Psychiatry* 1992; **14**: 86–98.
36. Poutanen O. *Deprressio terveyskeskuspotilaalla*. Tampere Yliopisto: Tampere, 1996.
37. Goldberg D et al. Ability of primary care physicians to make accurate ratings of psychiatric symptoms. *Arch Gen Psychiatry* 1982; **39**: 829–33.
38. Davenport S et al. How psychiatric disorders are missed during medical consultations. *Lancet* 1987; (Aug 22): 439–41.
39. NIH Consensus Conference on Late Life. Diagnosis and treatment of depression in late life. *JAMA* 1992; **268**: 1018–24.
40. Jenkins R et al. Classification of mental disorder in primary care. *Psychol Med Monogr Suppl* 1988; **18** (Suppl 12): 1–59.
41. Larsson S, Lilja J. The attitudes to prescribing of psychotropics among physicians and the general public. *Sv Farm Tidskr* 1992; **96** (2): 33–7 (in Swedish).
42. Keller MB et al. Course and natural history of chronic depression. In *Diagnosis and Treatment of Chronic Depression*, Koscis JH et al. (eds). Guilford Press: New York/London, 1995; 58–72.
43. Sireling LI et al. Depression in general practice: case thresholds and diagnosis. *Br J Psychiatry* 1985; **147**: 113–19.
44. Sireling LI et al. Depression in general practice: clinical features and comparison with out-patients. *Br J Psychiatry* 1985; **147**: 119–26.
45. Larsson S, Lilja J. The cognitive effects of a continuing education course about sleeping disorders for physicians and nurses. *J Soc Adm Pharm* 1994; **11**: 173–81.
46. Brugha TS et al. Gender, social support and recovery from depressive disorders: a prospective clinical study. *Psychol Med* 1990; **20**: 147–56.
47. Russel DW et al. Social support, stress, and depressive symptoms among the elderly: test of a process model. *Psychol Aging* 1991; **6**: 190–201.
48. Katon W et al. The predictors of persistence of depression in primary care. *J Affect Dis* 1994; **31**: 81–90.
49. Sargeant JK et al. Factors associated with one year outcome of major depression in the community. *Arch Gen Psychiatry* 1990; **47**: 519–26.

50. Kivela S-L et al. The prognosis of depression in old age. *Int Psychoger* 1989; **2** (1): 119–33.
51. Denig P. Drug Choice in Medical Practice: Rationales, Routines and Remedies. A Dissertation. University of Groningen, Groningen, 1994.
52. Sleath B et al. Physician vs. patient initiation of psychotropic prescribing in primary care settings: a content analysis of audiotapes. *Soc Sci Med* 1997; **44**: 541–8.
53. Balint M et al. *Treatment or Diagnosis? A Study of Repeat Prescriptions in General Practice.* Tavistock Publishing: London, 1970.
54. Bashir K et al. Controlled evaluation of brief interventions by general practitioners to reduce chronic use of benzodiazepines. *Br J Gen Pract* 1994; **44**: 408–12.
55. National Health Committee. Guidelines for the treatment and management of depression by primary health care professionals. National Health Committee, Auckland, 1996.
56. Elkin I et al. National Institute of Mental Health Treatment of Depression Collaborative Research Program. *Arch Gen Psychiatry* 1989; **46**: 971–82.
57. Thase ME et al. Treatment of major depression with psychotherapy or psychotherapy–pharmacotherapy combinations. *Arch Gen Psychiatry* 1997; **54**: 1009–15.
58. Coppen A. Depression as a lethal disease: preventive strategies. *J Clin Psychiatry* 1994; **55** (Suppl 4): 37–45.
59. Wittchen H-U et al. Lifetime of depression. *Br J Psychiatry* 1994; **165** (Suppl 26): 16–22.

12

Ethical Promotion and Advertising of Medicines: Where do we Draw the Line?

IVOR HARRISON

Crystal Avenue, Heath, Cardiff, UK

INTRODUCTION

The nature and varieties of "ethics" have been described and discussed elsewhere, and it is axiomatic that in professional life one occasionally is obliged to choose between satisfying one's personal ethics and one's professional ethics and even, in extreme cases, the law. The title of this chapter is perhaps ambiguous. Some readers may expect ethical advertising to mean the advertising of "ethical medicines", that is medicines which may only be supplied to the public on prescription. In this chapter the term will be used in the context of the advertising being ethical, which means morally correct, truthful, honest. In addition, consideration will be given to the advertising of medicines generally, that is those available to the public without prescription as well as those available on prescription only.

The term "patent medicine" was formerly used to describe medicines sold to the public under a name registered as the property of a particular individual or company. A few such medicines were, or had been, the subject of a patent, but are now more correctly described as "proprietary medicines".

Pharmaceutical Ethics. Edited by S. Salek and A. Edgar.
© 2002 John Wiley & Sons, Ltd.

Since these medicines can be sold to the public without prescription, they are also referred to as "OTC" (over the counter) medicines.

Until the 1950s most medicines prescribed by doctors in the UK were made extemporaneously to the formula given either in one of the pharmacopoeias or codices, or devised by the doctor. Pharmaceutical companies made "galenicals" such as tinctures and extracts of vegetable drugs, tablets, creams, ointments, for sale to pharmacies and hospitals for use in dispensing. Some companies also made proprietary medicines usually for sale to the public. Consequently, the companies had little need to advertise products to physicians. The multinational research-based pharmaceutical industry as we know it today did not exist.

The advertising of medicines involves two industries, the pharmaceutical industry responsible for the discovery, development, manufacture, packaging, distribution and promotion of the products and the advertising industry that advises the manufacturer on advertising campaigns. Both industries have their Codes of Advertising Practice, which to a large extent overlap.

In terms of turnover, the advertising industry is probably the largest industry in the country. Not only do manufacturers advertise their products, but charities, government departments, universities and the providers of countless services spend part (sometimes a considerable part) of their income on promoting their activities and keeping their name in the public eye. Even the numerous industry watchdogs regularly advertise, and some religious groups also find it beneficial to advertise. Why do so many different types of organization choose to spend so much money on advertising? The answer is the need to ensure that the public is aware that their service or product is available, although not invariably, advertisers also want to point out the advantages of their products to create a demand for it or to increase its market share. In a competitive world, advertising is ubiquitous because it is essential for survival.

Advertising takes a multitude of forms. The most obvious are billboards in the streets and public places, newspapers and magazines, and radio and television. While most advertisements in newspapers and on television are clearly and unashamedly advertisements, others are disguised as ordinary articles or programmes, often referred to as "advertorials" or "infomercials". Less obvious are everyday items such as pens, which bear the name of a company or product. Some members of the public can also be persuaded to buy such articles as tee shirts that advertise some product. Some people can even be persuaded to advertise their affluence by wearing expensive clothing clearly labelled on the outside with the designer's name or logo.

Ethics and morals are linked to law. In fact, in many countries, the law is based upon and reflects the predominant religious beliefs of the state. The law can be regarded as the expression of the minimum standards of acceptable behaviour. Since the advertising of medicines is controlled by law, it will be necessary to examine the legal constraints before considering the ethical controls.

It has long been necessary to impose some controls over the content of advertisements. Thus laws were made to protect the public from fraud. In the case of advertisements relating to medicines and medical and surgical appliances, the law also aimed to protect the gullible from harm. Unfortunately, such laws were only partially successful, and it has sometimes proved impossible to persuade a jury to convict. In recent years increasing reliance has been placed on codes of practice. Such codes have been compiled by a variety of organizations, often bodies representative of manufacturers of a class of merchandise, or of advertising practitioners. Until comparatively recently, most professions considered it unprofessional for their members to advertise their services to the public. Today, however, the majority permit such advertisements provided that they are restrained in tone and do not draw invidious distinctions between members. The limits are often incorporated into the profession's code of ethics. This is another interpretation of the phrase "ethical advertising". From the point of view of a profession or a trade group, there are two advantages to including some statement as to advertising in a code. In the first case, the content of a code must have been agreed by the group itself. It therefore has the cachet of being the collective view of the minimal standard acceptable to the group. The second advantage is that the enforcement of the code lies with the group. Alleged infringements are considered by the profession's or group's disciplinary body. There are at least two views about this. The groups would argue that such a body has a better understanding of the intricacies of the case than a group of lay persons acting as a jury in court. Consumer groups, on the other hand, would argue that the members of the disciplinary body have a vested interest in supporting their colleague. There is considerable debate as to which form of control is the best. There is a widespread belief that codes favour the advertiser because the sanctions available appear less onerous than possible legal sanctions such as heavy fines. Opponents to this view point to the difficulties of securing convictions in criminal courts and also to the delays before cases come to court. Insofar as medicines are concerned, at present both types of control are used.

While it is unnecessary here to describe in detail the legal controls over advertisements generally, a brief description of those relating to pharmaceuticals and similar products is required because they constitute the minimum standards applicable to such advertisements. Obviously, an unlawful advertisement would also be unethical.

DEVELOPMENT OF LEGAL CONTROLS OVER THE ADVERTISING OF MEDICINES

In 1912 the House of Commons set up a Select Committee on Patent Medicines to investigate all aspects of the trade in such medicines and the extent to which they were controlled by law. Its report, published in August 1914, made it clear that the law was inadequate. Many of these medicines were "secret remedies", i.e. made to a formula known only to the manufacturer. The Committee made a number of excellent recommendations, especially in relation to the advertising of medicines. It recommended that advertisements relating to "cures" for diseases such as cancer, diabetes, tuberculosis, paralysis, Bright's disease, fits, epilepsy, locomotor ataxy, venereal diseases and sexual weakness be prohibited. Moreover, "advertisements likely to suggest that a medicine is an abortifacient be prohibited". In addition, it should be made unlawful to issue advertisements inviting sufferers from any ailment to correspond with the vendor of a remedy, or to include fictitious testimonials. Several other recommendations would also have been of great benefit to the British public (see the Report from the Select Committee on Patent Medicines 1914, pp. xxvii–xxviii). Unfortunately, the First World War began on the day that the Report was published, so we had to wait until 1968 for the implementation of most of its recommendations.

However, a little progress was slowly made. The Venereal Diseases Act 1917 prohibited the sale and advertisement of cures for the diseases and also prohibited their treatment except by medical practitioners. The Cancer Act 1939 prohibited advertisements relating to any product or article in terms calculated to lead to its use in the treatment or prevention of cancer.

The Pharmacy & Medicines Act 1941 finally prohibited the sale of "secret remedies" by requiring all medicines to be labelled with details of their composition. It also prohibited the advertising of products for the treatment of Bright's disease, epilepsy, tuberculosis, etc., as suggested by the Select Committee, and made unlawful the advertising of abortifacients.

The Medicines Act 1968 and regulations made thereunder provided more comprehensive controls over the advertising of medicines to the public and, for the first time in the UK, the content of advertisements for medicines directed to practitioners was controlled.

Although advertisements relating to medicines are subject to control under the Trade Descriptions Act 1968 and the Control of Misleading Advertisements Regulations 1988, these will not be discussed here.

CURRENT LEGAL CONTROLS OVER THE ADVERTISING OF MEDICINES

The sources of UK law relating to the advertising of medicines are the Medicines Act 1968, sections 92–97 and regulations made under this Act. The requirements of the above are compatible with the current European law on the advertising of medicines as stated in Council Directive 92/28/ EEC. Since European legislation takes precedence over national in cases of conflict, it is convenient to examine the European requirements.

Directive 92/28/EEC

The Directive is divided into four chapters.

Chapter 1 sets out the scope, definitions and general principles of the Directive. "Advertising" is defined to include any form of door-to-door information, canvassing activity or inducement designed to promote the prescription, supply, sale or consumption of a medicinal product. It shall include in particular:

- the advertising of medicinal products to the public;
- the advertising of medicinal products to persons qualified to prescribe or supply them;
- visits by sales representatives to persons qualified to prescribe medicinal products;
- the supply of samples;
- the provision of inducements to prescribe or supply medicinal products by the gift, offer or promise of any bonus or benefit, whether in money or in kind, except when their intrinsic value is minimal;
- sponsorship of promotional meetings attended by persons qualified to prescribe or supply medicinal products;
- sponsorship of scientific congresses attended by persons qualified to prescribe or supply medicinal products and in particular payment of their travelling and accommodation expenses in connection therewith (Art. 1(3)).

The Directive does NOT cover:

- labelling and package leaflets which are controlled under Directive 92/ 27/EEC;
- correspondence needed to answer a specific question;

- factual informative announcements regarding pack changes, adverse drug reactions, trade catalogues, etc. containing no product claims;
- statements relating to health or disease containing NO reference to medicinal products (Art. 1(4)).

The advertising of unauthorized (i.e. unlicensed) medicines is prohibited (Art. 2(1)). Medicines need a marketing authorization before they can be sold. Such an authorization contains a "summary of product characteristics" (SmPC), which contains among other important matters details of the indications and uses for which the product can legally be advertised. All advertisements, including statements made by the company's salespersons to health professionals, must be compatible with that summary (Art. 2(2)).

When the marketing authorization is issued, that fact and the SmPC are published in the Official Journal and are therefore in the public domain.

In addition, advertisements must encourage rational use of the products, avoid exaggeration of their properties and must not mislead (Art. 2(3)).

Chapter 2 of the Directive consists of three articles and controls advertisements aimed at the general public. Article 3 prohibits the advertising to the public of medicines that are available only on prescription, and of those containing psychotropic or narcotic substances controlled under the international conventions. Only medicines designed and intended for use without the intervention of a physician may be advertised to the public, but none of the therapeutic indications specified in Art. 3(2) may be mentioned in the advertisement. The indications specified include tuberculosis, sexually transmitted diseases, cancer, chronic insomnia and diabetes.

The direct distribution of medicines to the public for promotional purposes is prohibited, but may be authorized for other purposes (Art. 3(6)).

Advertisements aimed at the public must be so set out that they are clearly advertisements, therefore "infomercials" and "advertorials" are banned. Moreover, each advertisement must contain, as a minimum, the name of the product (and if the product has only one active ingredient, its common name), the directions for use, and a clear, legible invitation to read the instructions on any package leaflet or outer packaging (Art. 4).

Article 5 of the Directive contains a lengthy list of material that should not be used in advertisements directed to the public. These include a ban on the use in advertisements of suggestions that a medical consultation or surgical operation is unnecessary, or suggesting treatment by post. Nor should advertisements purport to guarantee the effects of the product or suggest that it has no side-effects, or that it is superior or equivalent to another treatment or product, or that the product will enhance a person's health. There is also a ban on advertisements directed exclusively or principally at children, and recommendations by unqualified celebrities. In addition, advertisements should not suggest that a medicine is a foodstuff or a cosmetic, or that its safety or efficacy is due to the fact that it is "natural".

Chapter 3 (Art. 6–11) deals with advertising to health professionals. Article 6 requires that advertisements must include "essential information" compatible with SmPC and state the product's legal class. It may also state price or reimbursement conditions (Art. 6(1)). The term "essential information" in not defined. Article 7 requires all information given in an advertisement to be up-to-date, verifiable, accurate and sufficiently complete to permit the reader to assess the therapeutic value of the product. All quotations, graphs and the like taken from medical or scientific journals must be faithfully reproduced and referenced. All promotional material must state date of issue or revision.

Sales representatives must be adequately trained and knowledgeable about products and have available SmPCs for products discussed. They must also transmit to companies' scientific services any adverse drug reactions or other relevant information reported to them (Art. 8).

Article 9 deals with the question of gifts and benefits offered or promised to health professionals. The Directive insists that only those which are "inexpensive" and "relevant to professional practice" are allowed. It also states that health professionals should not solicit gifts, etc. Existing trade practices, e.g. discounts, are exempted from control.

Similarly, hospitality at sales promotions and professional meetings is permitted if it is both reasonable in level, and secondary to the main purpose of the meeting. However, it should not be extended to persons other than health professionals, such as spouses (Art. 9(2) & 10).

The giving of free samples of medicinal products to prescribers is subject to control under Article 11. Essentially, the prescriber must provide a written request, signed and dated for each supply, and there is a limit on the amount of each product that can be supplied. The supplier keeps a record of supplies. The sample pack is identical to the smallest sales pack, but must be marked "Free medical sample—not for resale", and an SmPC is sent with it. The supply of samples of psychotropic or narcotic products is prohibited, and each member state may restrict samples of other products.

Most member states already had legal or administrative procedures to prohibit advertisements that did not comply with the Directive. Insofar as the UK was concerned, a novel feature created in **Chapter 4** was the requirement to "ensure adequate and effective monitoring of advertising" and provide for "rapid corrective action". The sanctions available should include cessation orders or publication prohibition, the publication of the court's decision and the publication of corrective advertisements (Art. 12).

Pharmaceutical companies must have a scientific service responsible for information on its products, and keep copies of all advertisements issued. They must also keep records of how, when and to whom they were disseminated. They must ensure that all advertising conforms to this Directive, verify that representatives are adequately trained, and comply with decisions of the authority (Art. 13).

Consideration of these legal requirements will confirm that most of the main complaints made in the past about the promotional activities of the pharmaceutical industry have now been addressed. Moreover, there is little that was not already included in the Codes of Practice applicable to the industry.

ETHICAL CONSTRAINTS

These are of several types. The advertising industry itself has codes that are enforceable among its members. These Codes of Advertising Practice are compatible with the laws and frequently are more comprehensive in scope than the laws. Their main disadvantage is that they are enforced among the members of the organization and the only sanction for non-compliance is expulsion from that organization. Non-members and recalcitrant members are usually reported to the enforcement body for legal action to be taken if the "offence" is a criminal one.

BRITISH CODES OF ADVERTISING PRACTICE

These are enforced by the Advertising Standards Authority (ASA), an independent body created by the advertising business. It has an independent chairman, who appoints 12 council members, eight of whom have no links with the business. The members act as individuals, not as representatives of business or of pressure groups. The ASA's functions are to investigate complaints made in relation to advertisements and to monitor advertisements to ensure compliance with the rules. The results are published as Monthly Reports. Where necessary, expert advice is obtained from scientific and technical consultants.

The Code has the support of about 20 organizations, including the Advertising Association, Newspaper Publishers Association, Incorporated Society of British Advertisers, Institute of Practitioners in Advertising, and the Proprietary Association of Great Britain. Representatives of the organizations constitute the Code of Advertising Practice (CAP) Committee. The Code applies to all advertisements except those broadcast on radio and television (which are subject to a similar code enforced by the Radio Authority or the Independent Television Commission), those published abroad, and those relating to medicines advertised to the medical and allied professions (these are controlled by the codes of the ABPI). The contents of premium rate telephone calls are the responsibility of the Independent Committee for the Supervision of Standards of Telephone Information Services (TCSSTIS).

The British Code of Advertising Practice (the CAP Code) requires advertisements to be "legal, decent, honest and truthful". The Code contains a number of general rules relating to these matters and to price comparisons, worth and value claims. There are specific rules relating to certain groups of products. For example, the Specific Rules for Health & Beauty Products and Therapies are described in Rule 50, while those relating to slimming are dealt with in Rule 51.

In the event that an advertiser or agency refuses to amend or withdraw an advertisement, the following sanctions may be applied:

1. adverse publicity in ASA's Case Reports
2. advertising space or time may be withheld
3. the agency's trading privileges may be withdrawn
4. other consumer protection agencies may be notified

Proprietary Association of Great Britain (PAGB)

This is the trade association that represents the interests and views of manufacturers of non-prescription medicines, i.e. medicines which can be sold directly to the public. The (PAGB) devised its first self-regulatory Code of Advertising Practice in 1936 and has revised it regularly ever since. Strict compliance with the Code is a condition of membership of the Association. Companies must submit all advertising copy and packaging material (such as labels and leaflets) to the PAGB before the advertisement is issued. This applies to radio and television commercials, posters, leaflets, newspaper advertisements, internet material, point-of-sale equipment, labels, booklets and any other promotional material except that issued in the trade or professional press. The copy is examined by a specialist staff of pharmacists and consultant physicians to ensure compliance with the Code, and companies are expected to submit documentary evidence to show the accuracy of advertising claims. Approval lasts for two years, hence advertisements are kept in line with current developments in medical and public opinion. Furthermore, companies must lodge a copy of the relevant parts of the product licence with the PAGB and all advertisements are compared with this to ensure that unauthorized claims are not made. Moreover, the impression created by careful study of the advertisement is considered, as well as that created by a more casual or brief exposure to the document.

The pre-publication vetting procedures used by the PAGB Code are obviously preferable to a procedure under which advertisements are only scrutinized after they have been issued, if only because they prevent the unscrupulous advertiser obtaining an advantage over his more conscientious rivals. There are many people in all walks of life who would risk a rebuke to obtain a short-term advantage, and this is precluded by the PAGB scheme. Perhaps the best evidence of its effectiveness was contained in the Price Commission Report Prices, Costs and Margins in the Production and Distribution of Proprietory Non-Ethical Medicines HC469, HMSO1978 (1978, p. 33, para. 5.18): "The number of complaints about proprietary medicines is about 0.2% of all complaints (presumably complaints made to the ASA) and the number upheld is less than 0.1%. The conclusion is therefore that the system of control is effective".

The Association regularly monitors publications in which the advertisements are published to ensure compliance with its requirements. The PAGB Code also controls the giving of samples, the organizing of competitions and other schemes which aim at encouraging the sale of medicines. The sanctions which could be used against those who fail to comply with the Code are those stated for the ASA, since the PAGB is one of the sponsoring organizations of the ASA.

The British Herbal Medicine Association and Health Food Manufacturers Association also have a pre-publication vetting procedure.

Independent Television Authority Code (ITA Code)

Under the Broadcasting Act 1990 (sect. 8, 9) the Independent Television Commission was required to devise, review and monitor the effectiveness of codes or practice relating to advertising. Sections 92 & 93 of the Act imposed similar duties on the Radio Authority. The ITC has published such codes.

The ITC has a Medical Advisory Panel to advise on those advertisements which relate to medicines, medical and surgical treatments and appliances. The Panel also advises on advertisements for toilet articles for which therapeutic or prophylactic claims are made. The Panel consists of representatives of general and specialist medicine.

Advertisers have to submit copies of both the preliminary script and the finalized version to the ITC for preliminary approval. The final version then goes to the Panel for approval. Guidelines have been produced for advertisers, and these are similar to those of the CAP and the PAGB Codes suitably modified to be applicable to radio and television.

The Panel also advises on veterinary products.

Case Reports

It is very instructive to read the case reports published by organizations such as the ABPI and ASA. It is clear that both organizations receive complaints from a wide variety of sources. A few of the complaints do not come within the jurisdiction of that organization, in which case they are usually referred to the appropriate body. The reports are quite comprehensive and one can be surprised at some of the complaints. Cases are brought which at first seem trivial, but which are treated very seriously by the panel. Other, seemingly more serious, complaints after investigation turn out to be ill-founded. These statements are not made to imply that the adjudicators are not doing their job or that they are acting capriciously. On further reflection, one usually recognizes the justice of their finding. The point being made is that there is room for debate as to whether or not an advertisement infringes the rules, even among professionals.

ABPI CODE OF PRACTICE FOR THE PHARMACEUTICAL INDUSTRY

Fierce competition between pharmaceutical companies (especially in the USA) in the 1950s resulted in some very poor advertisements containing misleading graphs, and phrases taken out of context and the like. In the USA such activities led to calls for the FDA to take action. In the UK the ABPI set up its Code and took action even before there were any UK legal controls over advertisements to doctors.

This was first issued in October 1958, a decade before the law made any attempt to control the advertising of medicines to health professionals. The Code of Practice Committee to deal with complaints under the Code was established in 1959. It is interesting to note that at that time the members of the ABPI made and sold "medical specialities" (i.e. branded products not advertised to the lay public). The Association's members had already agreed that the promotion of sales should conform to two principles, namely:

- that the accuracy and completeness of the information given are of paramount importance, and
- that the methods of promotion employed must be appropriate to the learning and professional status of those to whom they are directed.

The Code aimed to ensure that the principles were interpreted uniformly and consisted of six sections. The first dealt with general matters. It defined "promotional activities" and required that they provide a complete and balanced picture of the product, including side-effects and contra-indications. Clinical and pharmacological claims should be based on evidence and clearly differentiated from theoretical speculation. Among other requirements discussed in this section were that advertisements should not mislead, and that disparaging references to competitor products must be avoided.

Section 2 dealt with mailings and insisted that communications should not be designed to gain attention by subterfuge. All advertisements should state the "basic NHS cost". All mailing lists were to be kept up-to-date and requests from doctors for their names to be deleted from the list must be honoured.

Section 3 required that representatives should be adequately trained and should not offer any inducement or use subterfuge to obtain access to a doctor or pharmacist. The Code urged restraint in the frequency of calls.

Section 4 concerned samples, which were required to be modest in size and value. Products which should only be used under medical supervision should only be sent when requested, and securely packaged to prevent opening by small children.

Section 5 dealt with gifts and hospitality. Gifts were to be of relevance to the practice of medicine or pharmacy and of little monetary value. Likewise, hospitality had to be moderate.

Section 6 insisted that information and advice on personal medical matters should not be given to the lay public.

Over subsequent years the Code has been amended and strengthened several times. Since 1962 revision of the Code has occurred after consultation with the British Medical Association and with the Royal Pharmaceutical Society of Great Britain. In 1967, the Code required companies to train their medical representatives in such subjects as anatomy, physiology, bacteriology and in therapeutic areas covered by their company's products. The representatives should also be examined to confirm their knowledge of these topics. The revised Code also required the companies to give additional publicity to the fact that doctors who objected to receiving mailing shots could request that their names be removed from the mailing lists. About 220 doctors (fewer than 1% of general practitioners) so requested. The Marketing Practices Committee was reconstituted under a Chairman from outside the industry and a Consultants Panel established to provide the Committee with expert advice.

The Code was last revised in 2001. It controls the standards of conduct required for marketing and advertising prescription medicines. There are really two codes, one for human medicines and the other for animal products. They are very similar and are published in the relevant Data Sheet Compendium sent annually to all registered physicians and veterinarians in the United Kingdom. Other interested persons can obtain a copy by writing to the ABPI.

The Human Medicine Code extends beyond the legal requirements and is drawn up in consultation with the BMA and the RPSGB. It also meets all the ethical requirements of the World Health Organization, the International

Federation of Pharmaceutical Manufacturers Association, and of its European counterpart.

The Code is administered by the Prescription Medicines Code of Practice Authority (PMCPA), which consists of the Director, Secretary and Deputy Secretary of the ABPI. The Authority also provides advice, guidance and training on the Code. The Authority may consult the Code of Practice Appeal Board on any matter concerning the Code. The PMCPA routinely examine a selection of advertisements from various sources issued by a variety of companies.

On receipt of information indicating that a company may be in breach of the Code, the Director will contact the chief executive of the company for comment. The company has 10 days in which to comment. If the complaint has been made by another pharmaceutical company (as opposed to a member of the public or a health professional), it must state those clauses of the Code alleged to have been breached and be signed by the company's chief executive.

After considering the comments of the respondent company, the Director may decide that a *prima facie* case has been established. The case is then referred to the Code of Practice Panel to determine whether or not there has been a breach. When the Director finds that there is no *prima facie* case, the complainant and the respondent company are notified accordingly. If the complainant does not accept that view, the case is referred to the Chairman of the Appeal Board whose decision is final.

When the Code of Practice Panel finds that there is a breach, the company is advised and given the reasons for the decision. The company then has 10 working days to give a written undertaking (signed by the chief executive) that the activity or use of the material complained of will cease at once and that steps will be taken to avoid a similar breach in future. The company must also provide details of actions taken to meet these obligations. The company must also pay within 20 working days an administrative charge for each breach.

Where the Panel does not find a breach, the complainant and respondent are advised of this. Where the complaint came from a pharmaceutical company, that company must pay the administrative charge for each matter alleged and ruled not to be a breach. The complainant is sent a copy of the comments, etc. received from the respondent, unless the latter objects that the information is confidential and this is upheld by the Chairman of the Appeal Board.

Either party may appeal against decisions of the Panel. An appeal must be lodged within 10 working days of notification of the result and must be accompanied by reasons. The reasons are circulated to the Appeal Board.

The Code of Practice Appeal Board and its Chairman are appointed by the Board of Management of the ABPI and comprises:

- an independent legally qualified chairman
- three independent medical members appointed after consultation with the British Medical Association
- four medical directors from pharmaceutical companies
- one independent pharmacist appointed after consulting RPSGB
- one member representative of the interests of patients
- one member from an independent body involved in giving information on medicines
- eight directors or senior executives from pharmaceutical companies

The PCMPA publishes regular reports of cases involving alleged breaches of its Code. In 1998 it received 144 complaints as against 145 in 1997, 102 in 1996 and 104 in 1993. Not all complaints became cases because occasionally no *prima facie* breach could be established. On the other hand, some complaints gave rise to more than one case. In 1998, 44% of complaints came from health professionals and 34% from other pharmaceutical companies (Code of Practice Review No. 23, Feb 1999).

CURRENT PROBLEMS

The laws and codes described above were intended to control the activities of those who made and sold medicines, to protect the public from misleading and extravagant claims. To a large extent they have succeeded. There are still some areas for concern, particularly insofar as advertisements to the public are concerned.

As has been said above, it is unlawful to advertise "prescription only" medicines to the public. However, as the recent launch of Viagra has shown, it is easy to evade this restriction. The company, quite lawfully, can hold a press conference stating that a marketing authorization has been obtained for the product and that it will be available on prescription from a stated date. The media then ask a variety of questions, all of which are answered carefully and truthfully. Radio and television reports carry the news to the nation to be followed up the next day by a variety of stories in the newspapers. Should some of these newspaper articles contain false or misleading statements, the company would not be responsible. The interesting fact is that the newspaper cannot be prosecuted for the inaccuracy because in English law it is not "a commercially interested party" as defined in the Medicines Act. A similar situation could arise without any prompting from the company. An alert journalist could put together a story from notices published in the Official Journal.

Another problem arises with the advertising of "borderline" products. These are marketed as foods, food supplements, cosmetics or perhaps toilet articles. Some such products can have quasi-medicinal properties, for example, a toothpaste containing fluoride could be promoted in such a way as to make unambiguous medicinal claims. If this happens, the licensing authority would require the product to be licensed as a medicine with all the testing and expense that would involve. While a manufacturer of such a product would like the public to know of the beneficial action of his product, he might not wish to obtain a licence. Clearly, he needs to tread a careful path when advertising the product. Some food supplements, such as vitamins and trace elements, are not licensed as medicines, partly because of the cost of obtaining such a licence and partly because any claims made would have to be substantiated. Such products are referred to as "nutriceuticals". Another way of evading the controls is to describe the uses and benefits in such a way as to avoid making "medicinal claims". Either type of product is often promoted by some "celebrity" known to the target group. For example, a prominent aging author has been known to write little pieces in ladies' magazines extolling the virtues of a natural product as a means of delaying the signs of aging. Sports celebrities are sometimes quoted, but more frequently these days shown, consuming a distinctively labelled container of some vitamin/mineral supplement giving the impression that they owe their success to the product. Neither type of product is likely to harm the taker, except perhaps in financial terms.

Public interest in medical advances is exploited by the media and often misrepresented. Today, "perception" is more important than fact! Distortion by the media is endemic. Ethical advertising needs therefore to take account of these factors.

PATIENT'S RIGHT TO KNOW

It is axiomatic that doctors should obtain the patient's "informed consent" before initiating treatment. This means that the patient should be informed of the benefits and risks of the various options available for the treatment of the condition in question. This has led consumers to demand access to a lot of information about medicines. In the European Union, the public has access to the Summary of Product Characteristics of each product given a new or renewed marketing authorization. This information is published in the Official Journal. For some years, patients in the UK have been able to read the data sheets for licensed prescription medicines published in the ABPI's Compendium of Data Sheets, available in many public libraries. Whether many patients derive any benefit from this is, of course, questionable. How many, for example, would know where to look for the information, and of these how many would really understand what they had read? The Labelling and Package Leaflet Directive (92/27/EEC) requires patients to be provided with a package leaflet or label giving specified information about the medicine language suitable. However, such a leaflet is available to the patient AFTER "informed consent" has been given.

In recent years a number of patient groups have been created to provide support and self-help to sufferers from various disorders, for example the British Diabetic Association. In addition to providing advice to the members and their carers, such groups may also act as pressure groups to campaign for services, or to publicize their special needs. They interpose themselves between the patients and doctors and can be of great value by "translating" complex issues into more readily understood language. Many of these groups have the support of experts in relevant fields of medicine and surgery who can advise on the value of new treatments. Almost all such groups publish a newsletter to keep members informed of developments. Some groups have set up web sites on the Internet. While all of this is very laudable, a few such groups, especially in the USA, have let their enthusiasm run away with them and engaged in activities which are unethical and may even be unlawful. Some have made statements about particular medicinal products that would have resulted in the manufacturer being prosecuted had the company made them. Patient groups commenting on the properties of specific products owe it to their members to be as objective, truthful and accurate as they expect others to be.

INTERNET

The Internet has had a major impact on all manner of activities; insofar as medicines are concerned, it has enabled researchers to publish their findings more rapidly and widely. Pharmaceutical companies, government departments (including regulatory agencies), healthcare professions and patient groups all have their own web sites accessible to all. Since it is easy to access web sites in other countries, users in the UK can obtain information on a company's site in say the USA, which the company could not legally publish in the UK. Clearly, there is urgent need for harmonization of legal requirements.

Furthermore, the general public is now being encouraged to use the Internet for shopping. All of this means that a wider audience has access to material than would previously have been the case. It also renders more difficult the monitoring of advertising.

Guidance has recently been published on the interpretation of Directive 92/28/EEC on the advertising of medicines on the Internet (*The Regulatory Review*, **2** (5), 26, 1999). It seems that publication of unmodified and unabridged versions of the SmPC, package insert, and the public assessment reports for approved products will only be viewed as advertising if there is some "hidden inducement" to promote the product. "Hidden inducement" is not defined, but would be considered on the facts of a case. In addition, "correspondence" in Art. 1(4) includes the exchange of electronic messages, but only if answering specific questions. Unsolicited e-mails constitute illegal advertising. The *Review* wonders whether this might be a move towards relaxing the ban on "direct to consumer" advertising of prescription only medicines.

CONCLUSIONS

No matter what form of mechanism is used to control the activities of advertisers, the "rules" will have to be written down so that all can read them. They will then have to be interpreted by those issuing the advertisement as well as those to whom it is targeted, and finally by those who have to adjudicate on the advertisement. It is suggested that unanimity in interpretation will seldom be achieved, not least because the viewpoints of the parties are different. Add to this the fact that the parties are unlikely to share the identical set of ethics and unanimity becomes almost impossible to achieve. It is also necessary to remember that there is frequently genuine disagreement among experienced physicians as to the value of different therapies for a given disease. Consequently, it is difficult to decide which to adopt in a given case.

13

Ethical Problems of Drug Categorization for Reimbursement

CHRIS GOOD

Thicket Grove, Maidenhead, Berkshire, UK

As Sir William Osler, the father of modern medicine, said: "The desire to take medicine is perhaps the greatest feature which distinguishes man from animals". Alone in the wilderness beyond the rigid confines of modern states, people may indulge their predilection to take medicines without any restriction save their ability to obtain the requisite ingredients. The conjoined paternalism of the modern state and the medical profession ensures that people are not allowed to indulge this desire without strict controls. These controls have themselves created problems with pricing and rationing. There is a tacit assumption in making certain medicines only available on prescription that the state and doctor know better than the patient what is best for that patient. This assumes that the state committees and doctors are adequately educated, a big presumption. It also assumes that all diseases have been discovered and named and their aetiology is known. Such pompous paternalism is obviously absurd. It is clear from recent history that there are still many diseases to be discovered and that existing diseases may have a new aetiology, e.g. peptic ulcer and *H. pylori*.

Modern states have introduced two mutually interactive concepts for the protection of the public, the provision of state health care and the licensing of medicines. Prescription only medicines are generally available as part of free or reimbursed state health care. Non-prescription medicines are

Pharmaceutical Ethics. Edited by S. Salek and A. Edgar.

available to the public at whatever price they are prepared to pay. A free health care system introduces unlimited demand for the provision of health care against the restrictions of a budget tailored to other demands on the gross domestic product (GDP). Thus the state is faced with the need to limit the costs of health care. Although only around 10% of the health care budget is spent on prescription medicines, the pharmaceutical industry is an easy and therefore prime target for cost cutting. A simple and effective way to cut the cost of prescription medicines is to restrict both the price of prescription medicines and those which can be prescribed on the state health care system. Another is to de-restrict medicines from being available on prescription only as soon as it is reasonably safe to do so, in order that the public may return to their earlier condition of paying for their own medicines. What are the grounds for restricting medicines to prescription only or general release? To understand this a brief review of the licensing of medicines may be helpful.

Since the dawn of civilization people were able to self-medicate with home remedies mixed with magic or religion or both, without any formal restriction. Gradually specialists in medical treatment evolved, variously known as shamans, priests, witchdoctors or quacks, and with them evolved the pharmacists who manufactured such medicines, principally from plants. It was the prescribing of remedies that allowed the so-called practitioner of medicine to charge a fee for his attendance and thus make a living. Unfortunately for the public, until very recently there were no regulations governing the provision of medicines to the public (1). From the beginning of the twentieth century the public had to rely on the rapidly expanding pharmaceutical industry, with its synthesis of active ingredients, to ensure that its medicines were effective and safe. Then came the thalidomide disaster between 1959 and 1962, with the birth of an estimated 10,000 deformed phocomelian babies in the affected countries. This resulted in the introduction of a voluntary licensing system in 1964 in the UK, one of the main affected countries, which was followed by a compulsory licensing system in 1971. Other Westernized countries followed suit.

Since the 1970s the sale and supply of all medicines have been controlled by law in most countries, the manufacturer being required to show that the medicine is of an acceptable quality, efficacy and safety. When satisfied on these criteria, the regulatory authority grants the manufacturer of the new medicine marketing authorization approval (MAA) for its sale. In the UK and several other Westernized countries, the sale and supply of medicines is regulated into three categories depending on the regulator's opinion of its safety. Those new active substances, whose safety has only been tested in a few thousand patients in clinical trials, are only available as prescription only medicines (POM). Those medicines that have been used on the market by a sufficiently large number of patients for the licensing authority to be further reassured as to their safety in the general population may be obtained over the counter from a pharmacist (P) without prescription. Those medicines which were in general use before licensing was introduced, or more recently licensed medicines that are regarded as generally safe for use by the public without restriction, may be obtained over the counter (OTC) with no more control than applies to other consumables. The various countries have different ways in which they categorize different medicines between these three categories. Controlled drugs are those liable to abuse or addiction and are always restricted to supply only on prescription. Their prescription is regulated by the Misuse of Drugs Regulations 1985 in the UK.

A recent attempt to limit the potential for toxicity in overdose is to restrict consumption with a limited pack size, e.g. paracetamol is now only available OTC in small blister packs of 36 tablets. Since the change in pack size, the number of attempted suicides by overdoses has fallen. However, this does not stop the carefully planned suicide who can build up and hoard an adequate suicidal supply. It does allow the manufacturer to increase the pack price and make further profits.

In the UK and many other countries, there is still no restriction on what medical practitioners may have manufactured or prescribed for a particular patient, whether the intended medicine is licensed or not, providing that it is legal and in the patient's best interests. In this context a recent case is of interest. A doctor was reported to the disciplinary body of the country's General Medical Council by the statutory health authority for prescribing single vaccine in place of the triple vaccine MMR, advocated by the health authority. This is clearly a political attempt to restrict a doctor's right to prescribe and may presage further steps in that direction. Another example is provided by the growing claims by patients that cannabis relieves their symptoms (mainly in multiple sclerosis). The possession and use of cannabis are illegal in the UK and therefore doctors are forbidden to prescribe it, despite patient claims for its benefit. The clear ethical solution is for the state to carry out proper clinical trials to test whether it is safe and effective. So far the state has avoided taking this obvious ethical action. There are probably several reasons, none of which are morally acceptable. One is the fear that making cannabis available on prescription would make it even harder to control its illegal use. This is clearly nonsense, since heroin and morphine are more dangerous drugs of addiction and socially disruptive, yet are available on prescription although otherwise illegal. They have a much longer and therefore apparently inherently respectable medicinal use. Indeed, until the introduction of legislation controlling the use of dangerous drugs, medicines such as laudanum (tincture of morphine) could be bought by the public from pharmacists without prescription. Coleridge Taylor wrote his famous poem ''Xanadu'' whilst dosing himself with laudanum for diarrhoea.

The regulation of medicines has developed ad hoc and is based on a plethora of mutually supportive concepts: politics, economics, paternalism, information and greed, which give rise to contradictory situations. Aspirin is available OTC for self-medication in proprietary preparations, yet would be unlikely to achieve marketing authorization according to today's standards whilst newer, safer and as effective analgesics are unlikely to achieve a licence. The authorities, in collusion with doctors and pharmacists who wish to maintain their monopoly on the dispensing of medicines, believe that they, the father figures, are best placed to decide what is good for the public, their children. The majority of people accept this regulation because they are vaguely aware of the disasters of the past and fear that there is too much specialized information about medicines for them to digest and come to rational conclusions about quality, efficacy and safety. Both the authorities and the people are agreed that the makers of medicines are not philanthropists who wish to benefit mankind, but greedy marketeers who wish to make as much money with as little effort as possible. There is nothing wrong with this desire. Most people are driven by it, whether gambling honestly in the stock market, the lottery, investments or in other ways, or dishonestly in crime, but the public also wish to be protected from the adverse effects of such greedy behaviour. So laws are introduced to protect the public. Since the majority of the public are reasonably law abiding, they support laws against criminal behaviour. The Napoleonic code introduced early in the nineteenth century sought to protect healthy people against the unnecessary nostrums of quacks by outlawing the administration of medicines to healthy people. This severely impeded the development of clinical pharmacology, which is based on studies in healthy volunteers, in France until reversed by the "Lois Huriet" in 1989. Since the phenomenal growth of the pharmaceutical industry in the twentieth century, the public have sought protection from uncontrolled marketing of potentially toxic products.

This need for evidence of safety and efficacy is based on the scientific belief that evidence from studies of sample patients from the target population can be projected to the population as a whole. Whilst far from all people agree with this approach and prefer only anecdotal evidence to support their whimsical use of medicines, as Osler concluded in his 1913 lecture "...how crude and primitive may remain a knowledge of disease when conditioned by erroneous views of its nature" (2). And self-evidently the same is true of its treatment with medicines. How should medicines be categorized, what information should be required to change that category and which categories should be reimbursed by the state?

As mentioned above, medicines are generally divided into three categories by the licensing authority: POM, P and OTC. What are the grounds for altering a medicine from one category to another? Practically all medicines based on new active substances are first categorized as prescription only until sufficient information and experience have been gained regarding their safety. Whether or not the cost of their prescription is covered by the state depends on not only medical but also political considerations of their perceived personal and social benefits. Some examples may clarify this. The antifungal imidazoles clotrimazole and ketoconazole were strictly limited prescription only medicines when they were marketed in the early 1970s for topical fungal infections. They are now available OTC for the self-treatment of thrush and dandruff, ketoconazole being regularly promoted on the radio. Peptic ulceration was generally treated surgically when simple antacids failed to relieve symptoms. Increasingly sophisticated forms of highly selective vagotomy were practised by gastric surgeons to try and separate the acid-suppressing effects of such an operation from its considerable undesirable adverse effects. Surgeons made a good living from such operations, but the cost to the health service in terms of operating theatre and hospital bed costs, morbidity and mortality were considerable. The introduction of the H_2 antagonists in the early 1970s dramatically changed treatment, although it was feared that lowering the gastric pH would encourage the formation of carcinogenic nitroso compounds and that treatment would mask the development of gastric cancer. There has been no evidence to support these fears. The H_2 antagonists became extremely popular, so much so that gastric surgeons practically went out of business overnight, whilst the health service made considerable savings. That is, until doctors realized that H_2 antagonists could be used to treat most forms of dyspepsia and the drug bill rocketed. With these increasing costs and the passage of time, the licensing authorities realized that initial fears about the adverse effects of H_2 antagonists were unfounded. They reversed their previous reluctance to de-restrict H_2 antagonists and made them P products, saving the health service a fortune.

A similar re-categorization or de-restriction of the proton pump inhibitors can be expected now that they have replaced H_2 antagonists as the most expensive treatments for various forms of dyspepsia. With the general acceptance of Marshall's evidence for the pathogenic role of *H. pylori* in dyspeptic conditions, antibiotics have been added to proton pump inhibitors as combination therapy. So far the licensing authority have been reluctant to de-restrict antibiotics, no doubt for fear of further increasing the already rapid rate of development of antibiotic resistance.

A further interesting example of de-restriction of an expensive class of medicines is the moving of the non-steroidal anti-inflammatory drug (NSAID) ibuprofen, used for the relief of pain and inflammation, from POM, to P to OTC. In the 1980s, NSAIDs came under increasing scrutiny regarding their toxicity, in the wake of the "Opren scandal" which was claimed to reverse the arthritic process but whose successful marketing in the early 1980s was followed by its withdrawal the next year in association with 86 deaths. Ibuprofen was marketed by Boots of Nottingham. In a review of the safety of NSAIDs conducted by Professor Langman and his group from the Nottingham School of Medicine, ibuprofen was classified as being in a class of its own and the safest NSAID. The review was based on reports of adverse reactions to the Committee on Safety of Medicines, of which Professor Langman was a member. Following this review, ibuprofen was deregulated to P then to OTC pain relief. Thus those patients able to afford it were once more able to treat themselves with an effective NSAID without prescription.

There is good evidence that pharmaceutical companies themselves may resist changing their medicines from POM to P or GSL as this may reduce their profits. Recently an advisory panel of the FDA said that it had not identified any serious safety concerns with three allergy remedies and voted that these three medicines were safe enough to be bought at pharmacies and supermarkets without a prescription. Health insurers showed that these medicines are safer than many of the other allergy medicines already sold over the counter. The manufacturers resisted the move, saying that the health insurers were trying to save money (3).

Deregulation of a medicine from POM to P and OTC should be ethically acceptable if the decision is based on good evidence that the medicine is most unlikely to pose a threat to the health of the individual or society when used as directed. The individual is already allowed to decide on the management of his or her own health with regard to two well-known toxic substances, tobacco and alcohol, and with dangerous appliances such as the car. Each when abused can have disastrous consequences for not only the abuser but also others not directly involved in their abuse. Thus society accepts the right of the individual to take risks and this right should be extended to the taking of medicines without prescription, providing adequate warnings are given in the patient information leaflet. The problem of deregulation only becomes an ethical issue when the medicine is no longer available on prescription for those who cannot afford to pay for it otherwise. Any medicine considered sufficiently safe and also effective for de-restriction to P or OTC should remain available on prescription for such patients. This is usually but not always the case. In some cases the government health service prescription charge may exceed the cost of the medicine, but those who can least afford it are usually exempt from such charges.

At one time the British National Formulary classified medicines as A, B or C depending on the Joint Formulary Committee's assessment of the medicine's therapeutic usefulness. Doctors were discouraged from prescribing other than class A or B medicines and preferably only class A. Some members of this Committee were also members of the Committee on Safety of Medicines appointed to advise the government on the licensing of new medicines under the 1971 Medicines Act. Thus the prescribing of medicines already granted marketing authorization by the government could still be restricted by this classification. However, the classification had no statutory power and fell from use by 1976, although medicines which cannot be prescribed on the NHS are still marketed.

The system has now been reinforced in the form of the National Institute for Clinical Excellence (NICE), set up by government to advise on best medical practice. This Institute tells medical practitioners what therapeutic guidelines they should follow and which medicines they may prescribe on the National Health Service. It thus basically decides which medicines will be reimbursed by the government and which will not. It is difficult to understand how on the one hand the government can license a medicine as safe and effective and then decide on the other hand that it is not therapeutically justified and refuse to pay for it. There are many examples of medicines not being prescribable on the National Health Service (NHS). Sildenafil was licensed by Pfizer for treatment of male impotence. NICE decided that this use was not justified on the NHS. Strong protests caused NICE to change its mind and allow it for certain patients with a chronic underlying disease such as diabetes mellitus. NICE also decided that Wellcome's recently approved antiflu tablet did not qualify for reimbursement, then again changed its mind, apparently due to consideration of further evidence following strong political pressure from Wellcome. It is difficult to understand how clinical judgements can vary so rapidly on consideration of apparently the same clinical evidence. At present, NICE has successfully resisted attempts to get β-interferon listed as a prescribable medicine for multiple sclerosis.

Countries approach the rationing of state-funded medicines in different ways. In the UK companies are allowed to set the prices of new medicines at market launch themselves. The government allows each company to make a certain profit each year determined by its various allowable costs. If this limit is exceeded, the government is refunded and prices adjusted to meet next year's allowance. In France the price of every new medicine is determined by the government once it has been approved by the same government for marketing. This adds a further delay before marketing. Furthermore, not only is the price set by the government, but also the reimbursement level. This is similar to the old three-tier BNF system of classes A, B and C. When last checked, 80% of class A drugs were reimbursed after use, the patient paying at first; other categories qualified for 70% or 60% reimbursement, down to nothing for some products that might be very useful, such as urine testing sticks, but nevertheless did not qualify. This level is currently being reduced in line with the need to contain the budget and reduce French social security costs.

These and other cases raise the important issue of whether the state should limit its health care budget and if so, how it should divide its health care budget. Clearly it must limit the cost of health care to what it can afford. To do otherwise is to invite bankruptcy on a national scale. Therefore it must ration the amount of money available for all the different aspects of health care, including medicines. It must do so in order to control the insatiable demand for and expense of health care. But should the state be deciding which patients get appropriate treatment and which do not, unless they can afford it themselves? In an ideal social order, no such distinction should be made, but in the real world of practical socialism, there has to be rationing and expensive new remedies cannot be exempt from this. But should the decision be made centrally for all doctors and patients by one committee such as NICE, or should it be left to individual hospitals and practices to set their own prescribing policies? At present in the UK we have both systems, so that even those medicines approved for reimbursement on NHS prescription may not be approved by the local therapeutic prescribing committee as items to be stocked or dispensed. There is yet another level of control exercised by the government on doctors' prescribing habits. Each year general practice doctors' prescribing costs are analysed and compared in such a way that individual doctors can be advised that their costs are higher than average and must be reduced. This should have the net effect of reducing the average annual prescribing cost, since high prescribers are constantly being advised and disciplined.

It is clearly immoral to deny a needy patient the appropriate treatment on grounds of cost alone. But who decides what is meant by needy and which patients are most needy? A relevant example of this problem is provided by that company which was advised by the licensing authority to withdraw its anti-acne product on the grounds that the antibiotic contained therein was unsafe and increased resistance when used topically. The company's appeal to the Committee on Safety of Medicines was rejected on the grounds, amongst others, that acne is a trivial condition. This judgement was made by a panel of middle-aged to elderly men who had long forgotten the agonies immature teenage acne patients may suffer when having to confront the world with their disfigured faces. The appeal was taken to the Medicines Commission supported by the live testimony of dermatologists dealing with such patients daily, who pointed out that to such patients acne is no trivial condition and may cause suicide. The appeal was won and the medicine continued on the market. Likewise who is best placed to decide which impotent patients should benefit from sildenafil? Who is best placed to decide which patients require cosmetic plastic surgery to alter their physical appearance to be what they consider more attractive, whether remaining of the same sex or changing to the opposite? Who decides whether anorexic patients are social misfits or ill people?

Who should be treated on the NHS? It is a dangerous policy to limit treatment only to those considered deserving patients. Do they include those wanting plastic surgery breast implants, plastic nose jobs, or only heart transplants for non-smokers? If limited to those not taking part in hazardous pursuits, we should have to exclude not only all smokers, all alcoholics, all drug addicts and those injured during criminal activities, etc., but also all vehicle drivers and all those doing sporting activities.

Attempts in the past to withhold treatment from patients who abuse themselves have understandably produced an outraged public reaction. Wherein lies the moral difference between a person who smokes for pleasure and possibly damages their body and another person who races motor cars and possibly damages theirs? Both are highly hazardous but, to some, enjoyable pursuits. Are certain clinical conditions, for example homosexuality, any more abnormalities or rather illnesses like genetically determined mental diseases such as Huntington's chorea or George IIIrd's porphyria? The situation becomes absurd. It is impossible to draw a line between acceptable and unacceptable activities or illnesses. Health care and provision of medicines cannot be judgemental and dependent on following a centrally decided acceptable lifestyle. Who makes the rules as to who is eligible for treatment? Those in authority may not always be in the best position to decide.

Surely such delicate and individual decisions cannot be taken empirically by a central committee, which clearly has a political remit to make sure that state funds are rationed appropriately. The state has the right to decide which medicines are sufficiently safe and effective in specific indications to support its medical culture, and grant marketing licences accordingly. It also has the absolute right to determine how much it is prepared to pay for such remedies in the state health care system. Thereafter any decision about which patients should be treated has to be taken by the patient and administering doctor at the time, with the patient's best interests at heart. Only at this level can a rational and ethical decision be taken as to who may or may not benefit. As the September 2001 BNF (4) rightly says: "The prescriber and patient should agree on the health outcomes that the patient desires and on the strategy for achieving them". This is important, but recent issues appear to make no reference to prescribing costs. More importantly with regard to the ethics of reimbursable medicines, the March 1989 BNF (5) says: "It should be emphasised that cost effective prescribing must take into account other factors such as dose frequency and duration of treatment that affect the total cost", and goes on: "The use of more expensive drugs is also justified if it will result in better treatment of the patient or a reduction of the length of an illness or the time spent in hospital". Thus there should be several important factors personal to the individual patient that go into a clinician's choice of the best treatment for that patient, which cannot be decided empirically at a distance for all patients. It is probably highly pertinent to the changing state health care attitude to rationing of reimbursable medicines that this later clause is now omitted from the BNF.

A final ethical problem with reimbursable medicines arises when they are withdrawn from the market, for reasons unrelated to safety. The licence may be withdrawn more for political than medical reasons. What can then be done to maintain the continued prescribing of effective remedies when no longer available? It is not ethical to stop a patient's medication when he/she is well controlled on it. By special arrangement with the government and manufacturer, special supplies may be made available for named patients for a limited period until suitable alternatives are found or they can be weaned off the medicine.

Not all patients like going to a doctor or believe in their ability to help. Such patients may prefer to avoid medication or provide self-medication. Every effort should be made to deregulate as many medicines as possible and as quickly as possible. The evidence supports the view that patients can in general safely be trusted to self-medicate with a wide range of what were originally and previously regarded as dangerous new medicines. They are no more likely to come to harm than on prescribed medicines. The government should nevertheless ensure that the prices of such self-medications remain reasonably affordable. This deregulation should ease the demand for prescription medicines and thus reduce the burden on the state health budget. This in turn would remove the need for political bodies such as NICE and inappropriate decision taking about what can or cannot be prescribed on the state. Either a medicine is considered effective and safe or it is not.

However, regrettably, emotional arguments usually appeal more strongly to most people than logical arguments. Nowhere is this more true than in the demand for immediate availability of potentially new discoveries in medicine to suffering patients at "reasonable prices". There has been a recent demand for the provision of illegal drugs such as marihuana for patients suffering from multiple sclerosis, despite the lack of any convincing evidence that it is effective. There is much anecdotal evidence from individual patients who claim that it helps them, but no well-designed, placebo-controlled studies such as required by the Licensing Authority for pharmaceuticals before approving new active substances. This paradox is key to most emotional argument, which takes individual cases in isolation without regard to the wider population implications. The Licensing Authority was set up as a result of the emotional outburst in the wake of the thalidomide-provoked phocomelia epidemic. The public did not want unscrutinized medicines going on the market. They want well tried and tested medicines with proven efficacy and safety, especially when other effective remedies are already available for that disease. The conflict between emotion and logic becomes particularly acute with possible treatments for diseases for which there is no effective treatment. To be compellingly tenable, ethical decisions should always apply across the whole spectrum of activities. The ethic that to kill is wrong is a moral imperative. This is clearly not universally applicable without disastrous results. To kill is to extinguish life. Yet to kill plant life is generally held to be acceptable in order to sustain life, also to maintain order by weeding out unwanted plants or to provide building material in the form of wood, leaf thatch or bindings. To kill bacterial and viral life is also acceptable in an attempt to restore health or prevent disease. Indeed, in an époque devoted to saving endangered species, it is quite acceptable to eliminate the smallpox virus, malaria and tuberculosis. So the argument about the ethic of killing becomes progressively more narrowed to animal life, vertebrate life, human life, the enemy and finally those who no longer desire or deserve it. Somewhere along this slippery continuum people, for various reasons, desire to take an ethical stand, but it is difficult to maintain a steady stance on such a slippery slope.

So it is with the licensing of medicines and their categorization for reimbursement. Having subscribed to the state health care plan, patients expect it to pay for everything. People also want to be protected from exploitation by unscrupulous quacks or companies yet want to be free to choose what they do to themselves and how they spend their money. A classic example of this is the use of tobacco and alcohol. Most societies agree that it is undesirable to allow young children to purchase tobacco or alcohol so limit its sale to those above a specified age. Adults are allowed to poison themselves to death with both.

In conclusion, most people want to be allowed to treat themselves and decide their own fate, but they also want to be protected from the dangerous and expensive products of the unscrupulous. At some time in their lives they have probably treated themselves with their own remedies which have been passed on as part of family lore, from friends, through advertising, or their own trial and error. Such self-remedies may not even be classified as medicines, but are lotions and potions made up at home, purchased over the counter or concocted from plants. People usually have great faith in such remedies, faith being the essential ingredient in their continued efficacy, but there is little or no objective evidence for their efficacy or safety. There is clearly a need to regulate the medicines produced by pharmaceutical companies, but this in no way addresses the problem of self-medication with home remedies or inappropriate use of other people's medicines. What the state has the right to decide is which medicines are safe and effective enough to be marketed, whether on prescription or not. It also has the right to decide how much it is prepared to pay for such prescribed medicines. It does not however have any moral right to decide who can have them and who cannot, nor whether they are available on the NHS, if safe and effective. Decisions about which patients get what must be left to individual patient–doctor contracts, otherwise the state will be imposing arbitrary judgements inappropriately.

REFERENCES

1. Mann RD. Aspects of modern drug use. In *Modern Drug Use*. MTP Press: Lancaster, 1984; 597–665.
2. Osler W. *The Evolution of Modern Medicine; A Series of Lectures Delivered at Yale University on the Silliman Foundation in April 1913*. Yale University Press: New Haven, CT, 1921; 11.
3. US drug firms resist over the counter sales. *Br Med J* 2001; **322**: 1270.
4. Guidance on prescribing. In *British National Formulary*, September 2001; **42**: 1.
5. Preface. In *British National Formulary*, March 1989; **17**: x.

Index

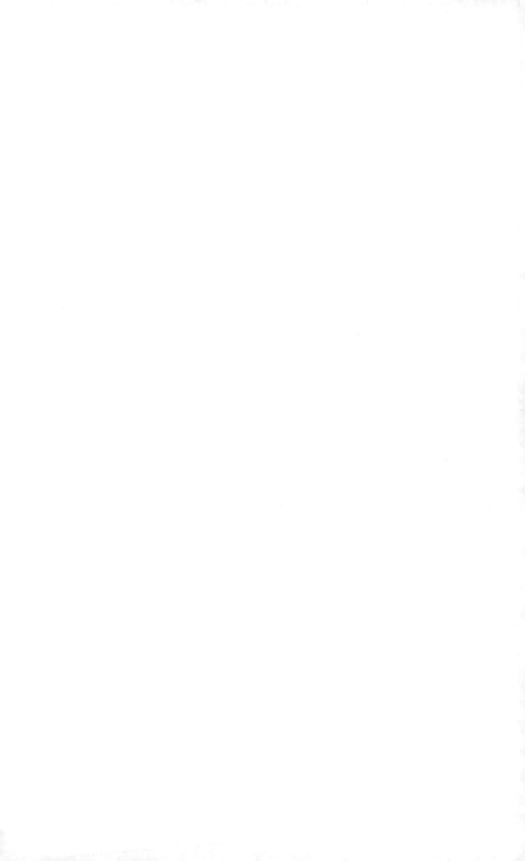